HOW TO LIVE
AND NOT DIE

I shall not die, but live,
and declare the works of the Lord.
Psalm 118:17

HOW TO LIVE AND NOT DIE

by

Norvel Hayes

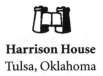

Harrison House
Tulsa, Oklahoma

09 08 07 06 05 04   10 9 8 7 6 5 4 3 2

How To Live And Not Die
ISBN 1-57794-724-X
(Previously published as ISBN 0-89274-395-6)
Copyright © 1986 by Norvel Hayes
P.O. Box 1379
Cleveland, Tennessee 37311

Published by Harrison House, Inc.
P.O. Box 35035
Tulsa, Oklahoma 74153

Contents

INTRODUCTION

God doesn't want you to have any diseases. He wants you to receive His miracle-working power and be totally free.

In writing this book, I'm doing my best by God's power to drive out and to demolish every disease in every person who reads this book. And the same principles taught here regarding disease can be applied to all critical cases—financial, emotional, social, spiritual, or physical.

Think about what God's Word can do for you while you're reading the following prayer.

Heavenly Father, I come in Jesus' name on behalf of the precious person reading this book. You know, Jesus, that I'm not a healer—but You are. Just within myself I have no power to heal; but Jesus, You do, and You live inside me. I claim Your healing and miracle-working power to flow from this book, like a river, into the body of the person reading it to drive out and destroy every disease.

And in Jesus' name, Satan, I bind you and I command you to take your hands off God's property, this precious person. I command this person to be free from disease. He has a right to be healed because he has been born again. I claim his healing to be so in Jesus' name. Thank You, Lord, for doing it.

And, Jesus, I give You the praise and glory for everything that's done, because we're a needy people and we need You. Within ourselves and without Your name, Jesus, and without the Holy Spirit of God, we are nothing. Amen.

1

GOOD THINGS COME FROM GOD TO YOU

You can receive miracles, and you can have authority over sickness and disease. Know this once and for all: all bad things that come to visit you are from the devil—all bad things! They come from hell—not from heaven.

The Bible says all good things come down from the Father of lights to you.

Every good gift and every perfect gift is from above, and cometh down from the Father of lights, with whom is no variableness, neither shadow of turning.

James 1:17

That means God sends good and perfect gifts from heaven down to you. Not one heartache has ever come from God. Not one weak day or one defeated moment has ever come to you from heaven. *God knows no defeat or sickness. Heaven knows no pain.*

I've been to heaven twice, and I can hardly wait to get there for the last time and forever. The air is full of peace. There is no sickness in heaven. There are no worms in the apples in heaven. The grass is about ten times greener there than it is on earth. You think you've got beautiful flowers here? I've got news for you—in heaven, those beautiful flowers never die. There are no seasons in heaven—no dying, shivering, or suffering. There is only life.

Everything in heaven is alive. Everything is full of life, power, and love. It saturates you all the time. Heaven is not a misty place out in the air, where a bunch of little spirits float around wondering who they are. It's a real world!

When you walk around heaven, you can see rivers, gulfs, trees, and mansions. And you can walk in on Sunday morning and hear Jesus preach! You think you're hearing good messages now, just wait until you get to heaven. Glory to God!

But right now I'm excited about the good things from heaven that we can enjoy in *this* life. Good gifts, perfect gifts are coming down from heaven, from the Father of lights to you.

2

FIRST THINGS FIRST—WORSHIP

Only after you worship and praise God, do you have a right to ask God to heal you or do anything else for you. If you don't know this, *it can cost you your life!*

When I tell people this, some say, "But, Brother Norvel, I love the Lord."

That's not good enough! A lawyer came to Jesus one day and asked him, "Master, which is the great commandment in the law?"(Matt. 22:36). Jesus answered:

> ...*Thou shalt love the Lord, thy God, with **all** thy heart, and with **all** thy soul, and with **all** thy mind. This is the first and great commandment.*
>
> vv. 37,38

In other words, Jesus was saying not to have any other gods before Him. He's supposed to be number one in your life. *And when you worship the Lord, you have made Him number one in your life.*

You can't love your church more than you love God. You can't love your family, your business, or your money more than you love God. If you do, you're in bad trouble.

Learn to worship God first. When you do that, you have a right to ask Him for anything. And He'll give you what you ask for.

One of the reasons why so many church people get in trouble with the devil is because they don't worship Jesus. You have to worship God *for yourself.* Just singing a song or two in church isn't worship. That doesn't honor God. If you run to church real quick for that, it's a wonder you even find the church. And one of these days you won't, because the devil will attack you so much.

Did you know the devil goes to church every Sunday? That's right. He'll help you sing, and he'll help you teach a Sunday school class. He'll sit beside you if you've got cancer and pat you on the back. He'll tell you, "You're a perfect Christian—don't change. You'll just have to die."

But, if you'll put first things first, there's no such thing as the devil killing you. He doesn't have the power to kill you, *if you'll worship God.*

You Can Know God, Have Power, and Still Lose Out

Maybe you've been a Christian for twenty years and know God real well. But realize this: the devil knows God. And he knew God real well, too.

> *Thou hast been in Eden, the garden of God; every precious stone was thy covering....*
>
> *Thou art the anointed cherub that covereth, and I have set thee so: thou wart upon the holy mountain of God; thou halt walked up and down in the midst of the stones of fire.*
>
> *Thou wast perfect in thy ways from the day that thou was created, **till iniquity was found in thee.***
>
> Ezekiel 28:13-15

In fact, the devil had lots of power. He went upon the holy mountain of God and walked up and down the stones of fire.

What iniquity was found in Lucifer, the anointed cherub, that caused his fall from heaven? "How art thou fallen from heaven, O Lucifer, son of the morning! how art thou cut down to the ground..." (Isa. 14:12). The devil started doing his own thing, going his own way, and that caused his fall.

*For thou hast said in thine heart, I **will** ascend into heaven, I **will** exalt my throne above the stars of God; I **will** sit also upon the mount of the congregation, in the sides of the north,*

*I **will** ascend above the heights of the clouds; I **will** be like the Most High.*

Isaiah 14:13,14

The devil's downfall can be yours, too. How? You could have been the best Christian in the world for twenty years and won thousands of souls to God. But if you turn your head away a little bit from Matthew, Mark, Luke, and John and start doing your own thing, you'll fall just like the devil did.

You could build a church of five thousand people and win one hundred thousand people to Jesus. You could be sharp and strong for twenty years of your life. But if you start getting settled and satisfied and start doing what *you* think needs to be done instead of what God tells you, you've had it!

If you don't watch yourself, even though you're called of God to preach, you'll get to preaching so much you'll just start floating along. One day you'll check up on yourself in your home and discover that you and your family haven't worshipped God in your house for four or five weeks!

You'll Get Weak and Lose Your Vision

It's easy for ministers to get that way. I mean, I have to watch myself. But, you can't afford to get so busy that you don't worship God in your house. From that time forward, you won't go anywhere but down. You'll lose your desire to pass out tracts.

You may say, "What do you mean, 'Lose your desire to pass out tracts'? I don't pass out tracts now!" No wonder God has you reading this book!

You'd better watch yourself or you'll get weak and lose your vision for getting people in your community saved who are dying and going to hell. You'll lose your vision for getting people healed who have cancer and are dying with nobody to help them. You can't help these people unless you know how. And sometimes if you do know how, you won't have the ambition to go and do it because you've lost your vision. Why? Because you've ceased to worship God every day.

So these people in your community just die while you're living right among them with the Holy Ghost in *your* belly. Remember what John 7:37-39 tells us:

> *In the last day, that great day of the feast, Jesus stood and cried, saying, If any man thirst, let him come unto me, and drink.*
>
> *He that believeth on me, as the Scripture hath said, out of his* **belly** *shall flow rivers of living water.*
>
> *(But this spake he of the Spirit....)*

He, the Spirit, knows how to get people saved, healed, and set free, and He lives on the inside of you. But, He won't do very much *for you* or *through you* unless you worship God. Obeying nine out the ten commandments won't give you an abundant life if you're not worshipping God.

Notice what Jesus told the devil himself:

...*Get thee hence, Satan: for it is written,* **Thou shalt worship the Lord, thy God,** *and him only shalt thou serve.*

Matthew 4:10

Verse 11 tells us what happened next:

Then the devil leaveth him, *and, behold, angels came and ministered unto him.*

If you don't obey God by worshipping Him, the devil has a right to come into your house and give you cancer. I'm warning you, the devil has the right to walk in and do anything he wants to do to you, *if* you don't worship God.

But, when the devil comes into your house and sees you on the floor worshipping and praising Jesus *every day,* he can't do what he wants to do. He'll leave you, too, just like he did Jesus.

Notice I didn't say "once a week," but "every day." Do you want God to come and hover over your house and stay manifested in each room? When you get up in the morning do you want *every day* to be exciting? God inhabits the praises of His people. (Ps. 22:3.) When you praise the Lord, you build Him a habitation, a dwelling place. Do you build God a habitation with your praise and worship every day?

Worshipping and praising God is a way of life. "Rejoice *in the Lord* always (every day): and again I say, Rejoice" (Phil. 4:4).

When Paul was getting ready to go to the Corinthians, they were talking about having power. Paul wrote them and said he didn't know if they had power or not. He was coming and, when he got there, he'd let them know if they had God's power.

*But I will come to you shortly, if the Lord will, and will **know**, not the speech of them which are puffed up, but **the power**.*

1 Corinthians 4:19

Some people say they have godly power because their services are good on Sunday. You can find out if people really have God's power by going to live with them for a while. Watch them every day and you'll find out just who has a form of godliness. (2 Tim. 3:5.)

Having God's power is a way of living every day. And you'll have God's power if you'll worship every day.

Here's how to start your day off by worshipping God. Bring your hands out from under the covers. If you can't lift them very high, just lift them a little bit. But open up your mouth and say,

Jesus, I love You. I belong to You and I thank You, Lord, that my name is written in heaven.

I worship You, Jesus. Thou art great, O God. I worship You, Lord. There are no other gods before You, Jesus. And I just want to thank You, Jesus, because You are my Savior and Healer.

Thank You, Lord, for Your divine, healing power. Oh, precious Jesus, Your healing power is flowing through my body right now to drive out every affliction, in Jesus' name. No affliction can stay in my body. I belong to You, Jesus, and I worship You.

Remember: put first things first. Only after you worship and praise God, then and only then, do you have a right to ask Him for anything.

3
GOD'S WILL IS PRAYING

After praise and worship, prayer is a natural step. *Heaven doesn't come to earth cheap. It never has! It takes prayer.*

Prayer is a channel that God has provided so that a man can reach heaven and see the things of heaven done on earth. *God's will is praying, not just thinking about something.* And wondering isn't God's will either!

The most important decision you'll ever make isn't whether or not to go to college and get a degree. It's all right to do that— I'm not knocking it. But it's a lot more important for you to learn how to *pray. Prayer isn't limited to anything.* If you'll learn how to pray and believe what you read in the Word, you can have anything you want. Glory to God!

When Saul of Tarsus was on the road to Damascus to drag Christians out of their homes and haul them off to prison, God stopped him in his tracks. Then God told Ananias to go to Saul, "...for, behold, he prayeth" (Acts 9:11). God sent Ananias because Saul prayed.

You may say, "The Lord would have sent Ananias anyway." No, he wouldn't because *it takes prayer.*

Churches need to get people on their faces praying before God for three or four hours. It would be good for them. It's not the Sunday morning crowd that keeps God's church growing and the love of God abounding. It's those people who come in during the morning hours and pray around the altar for two or three hours. They cry and weep until the Spirit of God floods them. Then they pray and pray and pray.

The only reason some churches have a building or get anything done at all is because of these prayer warriors. It pays to pray.

You may say, "I don't have time to meet with people in the morning and pray."

Then you'd better close up shop and take time to pray for two or three hours.

"Two or three hours? Are you kidding? I don't have time."

You'd better take time, you lazy thing. Remember that pride comes before a fall.

I know a church in Cleveland, Tennessee, that's been delivered from pride. That's right. The people go out in the field and pray for an hour before church starts. When the youth choir gets up and begins to sing, God comes and visits the place. The sinners can't stand it. They jump up out of their seats and run down front. Then they fall on their faces and begin to scream for help and mercy. Once the preacher never got to preach for six weeks. Why? *Because the people prayed so much.*

If you pray, God will come and visit you, too. Pray like a house afire an hour before church service starts. When your choir gets up to sing, during about the second verse, God will hit your place, too.

When the Holy Ghost takes a service over, you might as well forget it. Sit back, watch, and be nice. Let God do what He wants to do.

*If my people, which are called by my name, shall humble themselves, **and pray,** and seek my face, and turn from their wicked ways; then will I hear from heaven, and will forgive their sin, and will heal their land.*

2 Chronicles 7:14

4

GET SCRIPTURES TO
COVER YOUR CASE

To pray in faith for anything, whether it's healing for your body or a financial miracle, you need to know God's will. Then faith can begin.

The way to find God's will is to go to the Bible and find a Scripture that covers your case. For example, Jesus paid the price for our redemption *and for our healing.* First Peter 2:24 says "…by whose (Jesus') stripes, ye were healed." *Were* is past tense and that means we are healed. God will manifest Himself to you and your disease will disappear, as soon as you find out from the Word that you're healed. This Scripture covers your case.

Many people are waiting on the Lord to come and heal them *sometime.* They are trying to convince God to heal them. The price has already been paid, but you have to find the Scriptures that cover your case and make them a part of you. Never let them depart from you, regardless of the circumstances. If you don't do this, *you're whipped.* You will live your whole life without victory. It may even cost you your life.

Suppose you died at an early age from sickness. When you got to heaven, you went to church and heard Jesus preach. After the service you walked up to Him and said, "Jesus, I was a pastor's wife (or this or that), and my husband and I love You and we saw You heal lots of people. *But,* Jesus, why didn't You heal me?"

It will be sad, my friend, when Jesus turns to you, shows you His back, and says, "I did! Why didn't you accept it? Why didn't you take a long, hard look with your natural eyes at the stripes on My back?"

You may say, "Well, Jesus, I didn't see You on earth."

And He'll reply, "You saw that verse of Scripture. Why didn't you accept that as truth? It says that by My stripes you were healed!"

Attend to God's Word

Read Proverbs 4:20:

> *My son, attend to my words; incline thine ear unto my sayings. Let them not depart from thine eyes; keep them in the midst of thine heart. For they are life unto those that find them, and health to all their flesh.*

Pay close attention to verse 20: "My son...." God is talking to *you.* When He says "son," he means "daughter," too.

"My son, attend to my words...." *Attend* to them. Growing up on a farm, I had to learn to attend to things. If you didn't milk your cows, they would dry up. You had to feed the horses right because they would be working all the next day. My daddy used to check up on me to make sure I was doing things right. If I didn't, he'd get me. You have to attend to things or they'll just die.

The Bible is exactly the same way. God says, "My son, attend to my words...." That means *you're responsible to know what is in the Bible for yourself.* Quit driving around the country, wearing your tires out, looking for someone to pray for you all the time. *You* never walk the floor, *you* don't worship God or read the Bible very much. That's why *you* want someone to pray for you all the time.

Come to God on Your Own

You may think you've got to get to a particular person so that he can pray for you. *You don't need to get to anybody except the Lord Jesus Christ!* That's what you need, and it's *all* you need. Come to God on your own.

Recently I was ministering to about 2,000 people in Baltimore, Maryland. I was teaching on the importance of coming to God on your own and asking Him for mercy. While I was speaking, about 200 people got up and ran to the altar, fell down on their knees, and began praising God. *And all over the place God began to heal them.*

One lady had been pushed to the front in a wheelchair. After being shaken by the power of God for about twenty minutes, she arose from the wheelchair healed! *I did not pray for her.* She received from God on her own.

She came to God and showed great and deep appreciation for Jesus as her Healer. She reminded Him of how much she loved Him and how much she knew He loved her. And after God shook her like a tree, she rose up and walked off. Jesus said in Matthew 11:28, "Come unto me, all ye that labour and are heavy laden...."

You look up the Scriptures that cover your case, and *you* claim them boldly in Jesus' name. Go before the throne of God and remind God of what He said.

> For we have not an high priest which cannot be touched with the feeling of our infirmities, but was in all points tempted like as we are, yet without sin.
>
> Let us therefore, come **boldly** unto the throne of grace, that we may obtain mercy, and find grace to help in time of need.
>
> Hebrews 4:15,16

> **Put me in remembrance:** let us plead together: declare thou, that thou mayest be justified.
>
> Isaiah 43:26

Claim a Scripture for yourself, and the Holy Spirit will absolutely perform it for you. When you confess Jesus as the best businessman in the world, it's amazing how much money He will make you. He will help you accumulate things without much effort. He will show them to you. Put the gospel first and "all these things shall be added unto you" (Matt. 6:33).

Get the Word in Your Heart

Let's take another look at Proverbs 4:21: "Let them (God's words) not depart from thine eyes; keep them in the midst of thine heart." I want you to learn how important it is for you to know the will of God, how important it is for you *to not let the Word of God depart from before your eyes.*

The victory for you is in the Word, not somewhere else. *But you have to get the Word on the inside of your heart,* so your mouth can speak it. If the Word gets in your heart, it will come out of your mouth, "…for out of the abundance of the heart the mouth speaketh" (Matt. 12:34). Later I'll be emphasizing the importance of confessing right, but for now, you need to realize the importance of getting Scriptures that cover your case down on the inside of you.

You can tell what kind of Scriptures you need by what the devil is doing in your life. For example, if you want to live free from disease, confusion, turmoil, and other attacks of the devil, get into the healing Scriptures of the New Testament.

Someday *for your body's sake,* you're going to have to memorize healing verses! You live in a body and the devil isn't dead. Don't you know that the devil is going to try and attack you? That doesn't mean he's going to be able to do anything to you— you might be strong enough to throw him off. But the devil is going to try to attack your body, and your wife's and your children's bodies. You need to get that straight!

The devil is a crazy and ruthless attacker. He will do anything to get your whole family to die and go to hell. He has a one-track mind—he wants the grave for all of us. From morning till evening, then all night long, he's a ruthless killer. (John 10:10.)

If you don't smother the devil, you're going to have trouble all of your life. Even though you might be a Bible teacher, or a worldwide, well-respected evangelist, you can still get in trouble with the devil. He'll bombard your mind and try to get you to do things *the way you want to do them,* rather than the way God says to do things in the Scriptures.

5

DO WHAT THE
HOLY SPIRIT SAYS

"Submit yourselves, therefore, to God. Resist the devil, and he will flee from you" (James 4:7). *First,* submit yourself to God and obey Him. *Then* resist the devil and he will flee from you. Submitting yourself to God means submitting yourself to the Word. "In the beginning was the Word, and the Word was with God, and the Word was God" (John 1:1). God and His Word are inseparable.

Again, let me remind you of Proverbs 4:20-21: "My son, attend to my words, incline thine ear unto my sayings. Let them not depart from thine eyes...." To effectively resist the devil, you must keep your eyes on victory all of the time. How do you do that? By keeping your eyes on God's Word, because the Word is the book of instructions for victory. It tells you how to fight the enemy. If you don't submit yourself to God's Word, you won't be able to resist the devil. And if you don't resist the devil, then you will be doing your own thing the rest of your life. You won't obey God.

Don't Be a Rebel Son

Remember, "as many as are led by the Spirit of God, they are the sons of God" (Rom. 8:14). And the Spirit of God will lead you according to God's Word. The Word and the Spirit agree. (1 John 5:6-8) If you don't know the Word, you won't know if you're being led by the Spirit.

You may say, "Brother Norvel, I'm not led by the Spirit of God, but I know God and I'm a son of God." You can be a son of God and a rebel too—a rebel son of God! God has a lot of children who won't obey Him.

Often I write about things I've learned from God and done right; but a lot of times I've missed God. I missed God once in Atlanta, Georgia, at a convention.

The first day of the convention I taught on prophecy. When the Spirit of God came upon me, I didn't know what He wanted me to do. Before I got His leading, a man in the back of the congregation began to prophesy. He got me off track. When I got to the motel room, God let me know in no uncertain terms, *"You missed Me!"*

He told me He had wanted to bestow the gift of prophecy to various ones in the congregation. *I am the Giver of gifts,* He said. *And I wanted to give them the gift of prophecy—but you missed Me. You let that fellow prophesy; you let him get you off course, and you missed Me.*

I said, "I know it, Lord, and I'm sorry. In my next teaching session, I promise You, God, I'll obey You. I don't care what I feel, I'll obey You and I won't miss You anymore. I repent, God, I repent."

So, the next day the minister who had prophesied in the previous day's session wrote me a long letter. I read it to the congregation. He said, "Dear Brother Norvel, when I got to my room, the Spirit of God dealt with me. He told me that I shouldn't have prophesied in that meeting, even though the spirit of prophecy was on me. I know I was out of His will by doing that."

The Spirit of God had wanted to prophesy in that meeting, but the anointing was on me. This minister had the gift; *but sometimes just because you've got the gift and the Spirit of God is on you, that doesn't mean that you should get up and prophesy.* Wait and let the fellow up front either prophesy himself, or let him call upon somebody. You'd better learn to be led by the Spirit of God!

You Can't Do Just Anything You Want To Do in Your Church

When the Lord first began to use me in prophecy, He told me, *I want you to prophesy, son. But first of all, I want you to go and ask your pastor if you can prophesy in his church.*

You don't run your church. You have no right to do just anything you want to, even though you pay your tithes there. You don't have any right to override your pastor. God will not honor that. Your pastor is the head of the church (under Jesus), not someone else.

Deacons are fine men. As a deacon, I helped build a church. But do you know what we elders and deacons are supposed to do? We're supposed to sweep the floor and pay the bills. I know that deflates some people a little bit, but it's the truth. God's not mixed up. He called the pastor to run the church. God didn't call some man to run it who isn't even "called."

You and I are supposed to be good to the pastor. We're to make sure he has a good car to drive and new suits to wear, and we're to love him. When he wants to have a meeting, say, "Glory to God! Let's have one now!"

Don't stand around and be like some old, unbelieving deacon and say, "Well, you know we had a meeting about three months ago. It might be too early to have another one. Maybe we'd better pray about it." *No! Don't ever ask God whether to have one, just pray for revival! And then hold one.*

A powerful man of God with a highly respected ministry called me once and said, "One night I was praying, and the Lord told me to prophesy in services. He told me He was putting me in the office of a prophet. I prophesied a little during the next couple of years, but I really didn't know how important it was to prophesy."

He found out that when he held meetings in some of his pastor friends' churches, they didn't go for prophesying, especially when he would fall on the floor in front of the congregation and prophesy for forty-five minutes. That usually doesn't go over very well with pastors.

I brought this same minister to Cleveland, Tennessee. One night he was speaking, and all of a sudden he fell on his knees behind the pulpit. He leaned over against the side of the pulpit and began to prophesy. He prophesied for about forty-five minutes to an hour. The congregation sat there and looked at him. He even prophesied about the pastor's wife.

Now, this was a full gospel church, and the pastor's wife wrote the prophecy down, because she's real strict along this line. This brother prophesied about the price of gas going up and about other things in the world that were going to come to pass regarding the economy.

Later on, the pastor's wife told me that everything he had prophesied twelve years before in that service had come to pass, except for one thing. The other day she told me, *everything* has now come about. She still has the piece of paper, and she's watched it all come to pass. It took twelve years.

Believe God Scripturally

This same minister friend learned a valuable lesson in God the hard way. Once when he was preaching during a service, he tripped over a tape recorder. Right in front of the congregation, he fell on the floor and cracked his elbow, but he kept on preaching anyway.

After the service, his elbow was hurting really bad. The pastor of the church advised him to go to the hospital because his elbow might be broken. My friend agreed to let the doctor look at it. They prayed and started to the hospital.

On the way there, the Lord spoke to him and said, *Your arm isn't broken, so don't worry about it. I'll pay the hospital bill. And besides that, I'll talk with you about it later.*

My friend jumped. He asked the other people if they'd heard what the Lord said. None of them had heard a thing. When they got to the hospital the doctor said the elbow wasn't broken, but, worse than that, it was chipped. The doctor said an infection might set in that could result in his having to have his arm taken off. The doctor hospitalized him for three days to keep the arm still. My friend was really shocked.

At about five o'clock in the afternoon of the second day he was in the hospital, he heard someone walking down the hallway. The footsteps stopped at his door. He turned over in the bed and looked at the bottom of the door. He could tell that the person standing there was wearing a white dress or robe. When the minister looked up, there was Jesus standing in the door.

For an hour and a half, Jesus sat in a chair beside his bed and talked with him. And for all that time, no nurse or anybody else came into the room.

Jesus said, *You're wondering about falling in the church and cracking your elbow. You're wondering if I did it, or if the devil did it. So, I'll tell you now: the devil did it. But, I can also tell you that* I allowed him to do it, *because you've been out of My perfect will for over two years.*

You'd better not be mad at Me because I allowed this. (My friend said Jesus used the word *mad.*) *You were going your own way and doing things the way you wanted to do them.*

Now, read this carefully. Once you make up your mind that God is a certain way, it's hard for Him to ever help you anymore.

Most Christians have made up their minds and have their own approach to God. Almost every church in America, whatever their doctrine, believes their approach is correct. And God just doesn't bother them.

You make the decision about what you believe. God won't *make* you believe anything. You have to make a choice to believe

God scripturally. And, of course, when you believe scripturally, *there's no defeat.*

A lot of good Christians, who died before their time, believed God and loved God. Yes, they were good Christians, *but they didn't believe God scripturally.*

Everybody that is born again believes God. They love God and trust Him. And if somebody asks them a question like, "Do you believe God can do this?" they say, "Oh, yeah. I believe God can do anything." But you have to get Scriptures to cover your case. There's a vast difference between believing in God and believing God scripturally.

God's Word Is His Perfect Will

Jesus continued talking to my friend in the hospital: *You've been out of My will for over two years because you didn't prophesy when the spirit of prophecy would well up inside of you. You would override it when you were teaching because you love to teach the Bible. And I want you to teach the Bible; you are called to teach the Bible.*

But, *I told you two years ago, when you were praying that night, that I wanted you to prophesy. You did for a while, but you backed away because your pastor friends didn't understand it to that degree. You wanted to be friends with them, so you backed away from the calling that was on you.*

You'd better be glad that I allowed the devil to attack you, so that I could get you here flat on your back and talk with you.

It's hard for God to talk with a man who gets *his* mind made up to do things his way.

Now, you need to learn this. If Jesus hadn't talked with my friend, he would have died at the age of fifty-five because he had disobeyed God. For two years, God had told him to prophesy and he would only prophesy a little bit. Jesus told him that his disobedience would have cost him his life.

This brother was forty-eight at the time this all happened. At the age of fifty-six, he was destined by God to start a Bible training center that would eventually have an enrollment of thousands of students. Had he stayed out of the perfect will of God, there would be no such Bible school on earth. Years ago, God gave me the vision for the Bible training center he now runs.

Once I was visiting in the home of an Assembly of God pastor who lived in Indiana. While I was sitting there minding my own business, I received the vision from God. I opened up my mouth and prophesied it out.

My minister friend told me, "If the Lord had shown me that, it would have scared me. I wouldn't have known what to do. I had no earthly idea that God would put me in charge of a whole campus of two thousand students. I couldn't have believed that. I had made up *my mind* that I was going to get a room in a certain city and have about fifty people in each class each year—fifty chosen vessels of the Lord to be trained."

His wife had told me before that they were going to have only fifty students in the Bible school. After I had prophesied the vision, the minister's wife said, "Oh, no! I thought I was going to get to rest!"

I told her, "There is not rest for you and your husband. You know too much to rest. When you know God really well, you don't need to rest—you need to impart that knowledge to people."

In the hospital room, Jesus told my friend that many pastors die young, years before their time, because they pastor their church without ever striving to get into His *perfect* will. They operate in His *permissive* will. Jesus loves them, has called them, and they belong to Him, but those pastors will pay the price when they operate in His permissive will.

Pay careful attention to my words. They will help you today and *forever.* You must know and believe that God's Word is God's perfect will for you. And the Holy Spirit who lives inside of you will perform the part of His Word that you believe. He will perform it *for you!*

6

KEEP GOD'S WORD BEFORE YOUR EYES

I want to talk you into memorizing healing Scriptures in the New Testament and confessing that Jesus is your Healer. Don't worry about the whole world: first get things straight for yourself.

Speak God's Word

The first thing in the morning, I worship God. Then I confess:

Jesus, You're my Healer. You're the One who keeps me strong. You're the One who gives me health in my body.

And I will never have any want for anything, Jesus, because You are the best businessman I have ever met. All of my bills are paid, glory to God! And all of my businesses make a profit. Thank You, Lord, for thousands and thousands and thousands of dollars coming in above the bills, in Jesus' blessed, holy name.

Thank You, Lord, that my Bible school and my children's homes have no needs and they have thousands of dollars in their account. And that's the way it will be forever. Thank You, Lord, that because I'm going to give my money to help other people's ministries, men will give back to me again. You said it, Lord, and that's the way it is, in Jesus' name.

This is the Scripture I've found to cover my case:

> *Give, and it shall be given unto you; good measure, pressed down, and shaken together, and running over, shall men give into your bosom. For with the same measure that ye mete withal it shall be measured to you again.*
>
> Luke 6:38

Based on my confession, I believe that I will never have a need in anything that I do or that I touch. I will be *successful all the time.* My accounts are filled with thousands of dollars, in Jesus' holy name. My accounts don't run short.

If I slack up on my confession, my accounts begin to get a little bit low. Then I grab and shake myself and say, "Get your *mouth* straightened out, Norvel! This Bible school account has only a few thousand dollars in it. You'd better get your mouth straightened out."

Start confessing total victory in every area of your life, but first *you've got to get victory Scriptures on the inside of you!*

Don't Just Read—Study

The *only* part of the Bible that will ever work for you is the part that you confess and obey. The Bible never works for you by just laying it on the table beside your bed. It won't work for you just because you read it.

You must read it and keep it before your eyes until it gets in the midst of your heart, "for they (God's words) are life unto those that *find* them, and health to all their flesh" (Prov. 4:22).

Reading God's Word and keeping it before your eyes gets it into your heart. Then, when it comes out of your mouth, you'll have the power of confession on your side, because you believe what you're saying. (Matt. 12:34.) Until you get the Word to this degree, you haven't really *found* it. And the Word that you find, that's the Word that will be life and health to your flesh; that's the Word that you'll actually experience.

If you haven't *found* healing Scriptures, you won't experience healing life and power in your flesh. If you haven't *found* devil-casting-out Scriptures, you won't experience devil-casting-out power in your life.

When I gave my life to Jesus, I put a Bible beside my bed every night. I was going to be real spiritual. I was going to make sure that I prayed every night before I went to bed. And I promised God that I was going to read two chapters in the Bible every day, either in the morning or at night. But sometimes at night I would be tired, so I would read my two chapters *real* fast.

I did this for about a year. Then one day God came and grabbed me. (You need to be grabbed by God sometimes.)

I had just finished reading my two nightly chapters real fast, and I thought, *Oh, I'm a Bible reader. Boy, am I pleasing the Lord.*

God shook me right there in the bed and said, *Son, don't you know it's a lot better to study two verses and know what's in there and confess them, than it is to read two chapters and not know anything?*

So, I stopped reading so fast. You need to take it easy and *know* what's in the Bible. Study it, like you studied your school books. I mean *study* it.

Get Rid of Pet Doctrines

This may come as a shock to you if you don't pray very much, or go to church or read the Bible very much: Jesus *really* loves you! He loves you so strongly and so much that you can hardly understand it. He wants you to be victorious all the time, but you've got to find this out in His Word. You've got to get Scriptures to cover your case.

Jesus wants to heal you and bless you. He wants to save your children. He doesn't want them to go to hell. He wants to bless you financially. Some people identify financial blessings with God, and some with the devil. The Lord wants you to have *everything* you can believe Him for. He has provided everything *for you.*

Notice what Jesus said: "...I am come that they (talking about *you*) might have *life,* and that they might have it more *abundantly*" (John 10:10). In 2 Peter 1:3, we read, "According as his divine power hath given unto us *all* things that pertain unto *life....*" And 3 John 2 adds, "Beloved, I wish above all things that thou mayest *prosper* and be in *health,* even as thy *soul prospereth.*"

I have a diamond ring that was made twenty-five years ago. I don't have a lot of money in it because I bought the diamonds used. They're good diamonds, but used. Awhile back, I sat in a fellow's office who thought he was real spiritual. A person can get wild when he thinks he's real spiritual and get caught up in pet doctrines. I don't know how some people get these pet doctrines in their heads.

This fellow looked at me while we were talking and said, "Norvel, you know, I used to have a diamond ring like that, but the Lord told me to not wear it."

I said, "Well, fine! If you can't stand diamonds, then you should take them off. If my ring gets to damaging me, I'll take it off myself. I'm not hung up on *anything!*"

What in the world is a ring, but a half-ounce of gold? I'm not moved by people who judge me spiritually because of a half-ounce of gold.

You may say, "But I want to be just like Jesus."

Jesus walks on streets of gold. In heaven you'll be walking on streets of gold like He does. You can't tell me that God doesn't want me to have gold when it says in the Bible that He walks on the stuff.

> *And he carried me away in the spirit to a great and high mountain, and skewed me the great city, the holy Jerusalem, descending out of heaven from God.*
>
> *And the twelve gates were twelve pearls: every several gate was of one pearl; and **the street of the city was pure gold**, as it were transparent glass.*
>
> Revelation 21:10,21

The Holy Spirit Causes
Your Confession To Work for You

I asked that fellow who said that God told him not to wear his diamond ring if he could read. Sometimes I wonder if people can! They wonder if the Holy Spirit will do this or that.

The Holy Spirit will do what the Bible says and what you teach concerning the Word of God. Find Scriptures that cover your case, and get them on the inside of your spirit by confessing them. Then the Holy Spirit will keep you strong and the Scriptures will work for you.

If you will confess these Scriptures are yours, this is what will happen: When the devil decides to attack you, weapons will come forth for you to fight him with. He will have no chance to get you because the Holy Spirit will bring to your remembrance those healing Scriptures, or those on finances, or those on other areas that you have memorized. Jesus calls the Holy Spirit our Teacher and Comforter.

*But the Comforter; which is the Holy Ghost, whom the Father will send in my name, he shall teach you all things, and **bring all things to your remembrance,** whatsoever I have said unto you.*

John 14:26

When the Holy Spirit brings to your remembrance what's in your spirit, then it's your responsibility to boldly confess: *It's mine! It's mine! No, you don't, devil. You're not taking anything from me!*

Finding a Scripture to cover your case and keeping it before your eyes will bring you victory every time.

7

IT TAKES ONLY ONE
VERSE OF SCRIPTURE

It doesn't take but one Scripture to heal you. Find it. Stick with it. Say, "It's mine, it's mine! I've got it!" I know because I've had it happen in my ministry.

Many churches don't know what to do to get club feet healed. The ministers just pop the crippled person on the head and say, "In Jesus' name," and the person either receives or he doesn't. And that's the way it is, they think.

That's *not* the way it is. You can pop people on the head for fifty years; but, if you have club feet, that's not the way healing happens. You need to get a verse of Scripture on the inside of you. You need to confess it and call your feet normal.

Club Feet Healed Through James 5:14-15

One night, I was ministering these verses:

> *Is any sick among you? Let him call for the elders of the church; and let them pray over him, anointing him with oil in the name of the Lord:*

And the prayer of faith shall save the sick, and the Lord shall raise him up; and if he have committed sins, they shall be forgiven him.

James 5:14,15

I told the audience to pray the prayer of faith and to get James 5:14-15 to be a part of them. I told them they must do it. A man with club feet came forward, and I prayed and anointed him with oil.

I didn't feel anything when I prayed and anointed him. And as far as I know, he didn't either. All he needed to know, believe, and say was: "I got anointed with oil tonight in the name of the Lord. The prayer of faith was prayed for me. According to James 5:14-15, I've got new feet; and according to James 5:14-15, I'm healed. Because it was ministered to me, I've got my healing! I'm accepting it; I'm making it a part of me. Thank You, Lord, for healing me!"

I told him, along with the rest of the congregation, "When you get home, don't start talking with your wife or husband. I mean, don't hold a natural conversation with them. Go to bed and go to sleep saying, 'James 5:14-15 is mine! The prayer of faith was prayed for me and I got it! *It's mine!'*"

The man with club feet went home saying what I told him to say. He went to sleep saying it.

When I teach you something from the Word of God, if you'll do it, you can receive *your* healing and *your* miracle. If you veer away from it just a little bit, you're not going to receive anything. Get that straight! You either believe Jesus by faith, or you don't believe Him.

The next night in the parking lot of the church, a very distin-
guished looking businessman came up to me and said, "Brother
Norvel, I've got something to tell you! For years I've heard James
5:14-15 preached. I've seen people anointed with oil for twenty-
some years of my life. *But I never received until last night.*

"You pounded it into me; you taught it to me. You kept on
teaching it, *and I accepted it.* You kept on and on giving me
instructions in what to do, until I got it!

"I did exactly what you told me to do, and I began to receive
on the inside of me. I went to bed and went to sleep without
talking to my wife because you told me not to. This morning
when I woke up, I moved the cover back and swung my legs
over onto the floor. I wasn't really thinking about anything, but
when I looked down at my feet, *I saw that they were normal!*"

The man's club feet were healed!

Don't Live in a World of Talk
Not Based on the Scriptures

It's all right to talk to your wife, but not while you're trying to
talk to God. Talk to God first, then to your wife, and you'll make
a lot better husband. Don't go around talking to your wife
without ever quoting Scriptures. If you do, all you'll do is live in
a world of talk, talk, talk. Then you'll say things like this: "I
wonder why God doesn't do this. I wonder why God doesn't do
that. I wonder why I'm sick. I wonder why I've got club feet.
Well, maybe He just doesn't want to heal me, or maybe He's
using this for His glory."

Human beings shouldn't get glory for what God does. I was
just a teacher who very simply instructed on two verses of

Scripture—that's all I was. But because the man with club feet got these two Scriptures down inside him, God came to him sometime during the night with His healing power.

You can get so messed up talking to other people that you don't know what you're doing. If you want to be healed, don't talk to another human being—*talk to God!* Go to bed talking to God. Forget about human beings and go to bed with James 5:14-15, saying, *"I've got it, Jesus; it's mine!"*

Learn It, Believe It, Do It

I've been called to be a Bible teacher; I'm a channel for instructions. A teacher obviously *teaches.* For example, an evangelist comes in and holds salvation-type services; but a teacher's calling is to teach you about God.

I can walk into a room, open the Bible up, and God will unfold to me exactly what to do for a certain time. For example, He'll show me what to do for a crippled person. I can teach him how to have total deliverance and total freedom.

I walked in the office of a teacher; I teach a verse of Scripture. But *you* have to learn it. You have to *learn* what it says, and *believe* what it says, and *do* what it says. I have to teach people, day after day. It might take me days and days to teach them exactly what to say, and to say it *every day.* But *I can teach them* to talk like they're supposed to talk and to call upon Jesus.

I've had them calling Jesus their Healer and calling their legs straight. I've had them saying it *loud and strong.* It might take two years, but it doesn't make any difference. God will come to them one of these nights, and they'll wake up totally normal.

The man who had club feet believed James 5:14-15 and did what it said. He doesn't have club feet anymore. God gave him two brand-new feet. He had never run in his life. When you've got goofed up feet, you have to walk. But when he looked down and saw two normal feet, he got so excited that he jumped up, pulled his trousers on, and ran a mile. Thank the Lord!

I thought of Elijah, who outran the chariots and horses of King Ahab. (1 Kings 18:46.) I told this man that the power of the Lord had to have been with him, or he would have had a heart attack.

He gave his testimony to the church that night. He pulled up his pants legs and showed the people his normal feet. The whole church laughed.

Did you know that most churches don't even know that Jesus will come to you and heal you and give you two new feet if you need them? But He will. All it takes is getting one verse of Scripture on the inside of you and sticking with it!

Quit Talking After You've Said What God Says

A lady who attended a Nazarene church stood on one verse of Scripture and saw her twisted, deformed daughter made completely whole and become a worldwide evangelist. This Nazarene woman read in the Word that Jesus said "...If thou canst believe, all things are possible to him that believeth" (Mark 9:23).

So she *said* with her mouth, "Jesus, You said all things are possible to him that believes. I love You, Jesus, and I believe for You to come to *my* house and make *my* daughter *normal*." Then she never wavered!

The reason God doesn't come and visit some people more is because they don't quit talking after they've said what God says. The Lord was saying *only believe*. This Nazarene mother believed all the time; she stood on this one verse of Scripture.

Every person you know who is facing death before their time needs only one verse of Scripture to bring them total health. You don't have to memorize a chapter in the Bible to be healed. You only have to know one verse. It can bring you a total miracle.

This Nazarene lady knew more about the Bible, but it was one verse that brought her a miracle: "...all things are possible to him that believeth."

Many churches don't believe that a little waterhead baby can be made completely normal while in your hands. They don't a bit more believe that than they believe Castro is on the moon dancing with a pink apron on. The average church in America would say, "Well, yes, I know God could do it *if* He wanted to. Oh, yes, I believe God can do anything!"

Why, they don't either! If they did, they would stand on the Scriptures *all the time* and would *never* waver. They would totally refuse to waver!

Deformed Daughter Healed Through Mark 9:23

The Nazarene mother went on and on. Every day. Every week. Every month. Every year. She said, "Jesus, I believe! I believe for You, Jesus, to come to *my* house and make *my* daughter normal."

Her daughter was so twisted and crippled when she came forth out of the womb, that she had to be fed through her veins. Everything about her was deformed. And still the mother said, "I believe for You to come to *my* house and make *my* daughter normal."

How long did she say it? How long did she believe it? *She believed it and said it for fourteen years.* If you get tired at twelve years, it won't work. Just don't ever get tired.

In the fourteenth year, Jesus said, "Your faith has pleased me, and I'm going to come to your house and heal your daughter."

That's exactly what Jesus told her. Coming from her house, her faith had welled up before the throne of God for fourteen years. Jesus *heard* it. He *saw* it. For fourteen years, He was pleased.

The Word of God will get Jesus to manifest Himself by the power of the Holy Spirit. So on the day Jesus told this mother He was going to come, a little white cloud began to form in the living room. The wind began to blow around the house, and the cloud got bigger and bigger in the living room. All of a sudden, Jesus appeared and stepped out of the cloud. He walked over to the wheelchair and laid His hands upon the deformed girl. Her jawbone began to pop and crack. It became normal and straight and smooth. All of her bones began to pop and jerk. The little girl was made totally normal.

She leaped out of the wheelchair and began to run and jump with her totally healed body. Her back had been so twisted and knotted that the doctors at Mayo Clinic said it was impossible for her to ever be normal. Every knot on her back disappeared and her backbone was totally healed. All this happened because a mother confessed and believed one verse of Scripture for fourteen years and didn't give up.

8

TALK RIGHT

God's power is released the moment God stamps your confession approved. The power will come and give you what you've been confessing. If it's a blessing for finances, for your body or your mind, or for your children, it will come. If you're confessing for your children, God will come to them.

"What do you mean, 'God will come to them'? My children won't listen to anybody, Brother Norvel."

My daughter wouldn't listen to anybody either; but God sent an angel into her room about as big as two men and scared all the devils out of her! *But,* I confessed right regarding her.

Let me teach you how to talk. If you'll let me do that, you'll be able to teach your relatives and friends who need the Lord Jesus to do something for them.

Your World Is Formed by Your Words

The Holy Spirit will perform the scriptural words of *anyone* who *says* them and *obeys* them. God is a Spirit and God performs words. Your whole world is made out of your words. You put yourself in the kind of world you're living in today—

rich, poor, healthy, sickly, or whatever—with your *mouth*. I didn't say someone else's mouth; *your mouth* put you there.

Always remember this: *you are* your own worst enemy—not someone else, *you*. You don't have to pay any attention to flakey people who will get you all messed up. You have a right to walk with God yourself. You have a right to claim the Scriptures, the riches of heaven, yourself. And if you will do it yourself, God will come and visit you.

"What will He bring with Him, Brother Norvel?"

Everything that you can believe Him for and everything that you've been confessing. God always brings to your house and to your life gifts from heaven. Every gift that you've ever claimed (really claimed) from heaven, *you've gotten it!*

"Well, I haven't claimed anything, Brother Norvel."

That's the reason you're a total wreck. You just sit around and don't claim anything. The Lord Jesus Christ has paid the price and given His name and His power over to the New Testament church. The New Testament is a better covenant than the Old Testament.

> But now hath he (Jesus) obtained a more excellent ministry, by how much also he is the mediator of a **better covenant**, which was established upon **better promises**.
>
> Hebrews 8:6

The better covenant is enjoyed by people who learn how to talk right. I mentioned earlier that whatever state you're in today, your own mouth put you there. Your mouth, or your tongue, is like the steering wheel of a car. The car goes whichever way you turn the steering wheel. It's like the helm of a ship.

Behold, we put bits in the horses' mouths, that they may obey us; and we turn about their whole body.

Behold also the ships, which though they are so great, and are driven by fierce winds, yet are they turned about with a very small helm, whitersoever the governor listeth.

Even so the tongue is a little member, and boasteth great things....

James 3:3-5

The way you confess every day is the kind of life you will have.

*Death and life are in the power of the tongue: and they that love **it shall eat the fruit thereof.***

Proverbs 18:21

Thank God, I begin my day by walking the floor and worshipping God. Thank God, I've already started my day, today, speaking right things. You've got to stir up the gift that's within you and get your mind functioning right. (2 Tim. 1:6.)

A tremendously successful minister in our world today said one of the worst things about Americans is that they haven't learned how to live yet. They just do whatever they want. They get up every morning and just float along and let whatever happens, happen. And whatever doesn't happen, well, "That just wasn't for me."

Nothing *just happens* to you, unless you let it happen! When something bad begins to happen, bind it in Jesus' name and throw it out! God doesn't believe in your having sad days. He doesn't have any. God doesn't even know the meaning of blue Mondays, because He talks right and confesses right *all the time.*

I mean, if God wants a world, He says, "World, I speak to you, come into being." And all of a sudden, *there is a world.*

*In the beginning God created the heaven and the earth. And God **said**, Let there be light: and there was light. And God **said**, Let there be a firmament in the midst of the waters....*

*And God **said**, Let the waters under the heaven be gathered together....*

*And God **said**, Let the earth bring forth grass, the herb yielding seed, and the fruit tree yielding fruit....*

And God saw every thing that he had made, and behold, it was very good....

Genesis 1:1,3,6,9,11,31

The world was formed by words from the mouth of God. "Through faith we understand that the worlds were framed by the word of God..." (Heb. 11:3). Your body was formed and made by the words of God. "And God *said*, Let us make man in our image..." (Gen. 1:26).

All of the good things that you see here—the lakes and the mountains—were formed by words out of the mouth of God. And the same kind of thing happens to you all of the time.

Your whole world is formed out of the words *your* mouth speaks—out of *your* confession. There's all kinds of power in confession!

"What kind of power, Brother Norvel?"

Any kind of power you want, just name it. Anybody in the world can be successful, *if* they learn how to talk—*anybody* can. You can have anything you want from God, *if* you'll learn how to talk!

"What do you mean *talk?*"

I don't mean the natural kind of talking; almost anyone can hold a conversation. I'm talking about looking up Scriptures that apply to your life, Scriptures that you really need, *Scriptures that cover your case,* and getting them on the inside of you, so you can talk right.

9

CONFESSION BRINGS
YOU POSSESSION

Once I was in Canada speaking at a small church, and the Lord started dealing with me to teach the people how to talk. I had no earthly idea that learning how to talk could be so powerful and *so important.*

Jesus thought it was very important to talk right. In Matthew 21:21 He said, "...if ye shall say unto this mountain, Be thou removed, and be thou cast into the sea, it shall be done."

That day I used this Scripture and taught *Confession Brings You Possession.* After I spoke, I gave an altar call that dealt along the same line. The Spirit of God was working pretty strong. So when I gave the invitation, about forty or fifty people came forward. Someone pushed a man in a wheelchair down the aisle. I'd never heard any minister in the world tell someone what the Holy Spirit was about to have me tell this man in the wheelchair. And I'd never seen anyone minister to someone like I was about to minister to him.

(It's amazing how much smarter God is than you or me. If you just listen to yourself, you'll think you have a lot of sense; especially if you've been preaching or reading the Bible for a long time. Let me pass this on to you: you'll never know just how dumb you are until you get to heaven! And the same goes for me, too.)

As the man came rolling down the aisle, I yelled, "Confession brings you possession!" As I said this, the word of the Lord came unto me saying, *What you taught will work for him, if he will obey it! Now, son, I want you to point out that there are* if's *in there. Turn in your Bible to Matthew 21 and point out the* if's *to the people. Point out the* if's *so they can see for themselves.*

I'd never heard anything like that in my life at any gospel service. So I said, "Is that right? Glory to God! It will work for him, *if* he will obey it."

In verse 21, Jesus tells us what the if's are:

> ...*Verily I say unto you, If ye (talking about **you**) have faith, and doubt not....*

God doesn't want you to doubt. He works with your faith. God is a faith God.

If You're Ashamed, You Don't Believe

> ...*If ye have faith, and doubt not, ye (not somebody else for you) shall not only do this which is done to the fig tree, but also if...*
> Matthew 21:21

But also *if* means believe and doubt not. Realize this: You don't believe if you're ashamed to run a big ad in your hometown newspaper in bold letters, saying, "We are going to have a healing service on Sunday night and Jesus is going to heal people in our church. Bring the sick and the demon-possessed so Jesus can heal them."

If you're the pastor and you're ashamed to put your church name and your name in this ad, that means you don't believe! You only think you believe. And you'll never be able to believe God to do things for you, until you get rid of some of those religious ideas of yours or your relatives. *Never!*

The Bible says, "If the Son, therefore, shall make you free, ye shall be free indeed" (John 8:36). Jesus has paid the price for you to be free. He wants you to open your mind, your spirit, and your entire being to God and believe God for anything. Believe God boldly!

"But, Brother Norvel, I don't have very many friends who believe like that!"

Who cares what your friends believe? God says for you to get delivered from your friends and your relatives. If you can believe it, He will do great things for you. It's amazing what He will do for you, but you need to have faith. Anything you're holding back and making excuses for, that's doubt and unbelief and God won't work through it.

You say, "Well, don't you believe that God would still do such-and-such in these conditions and this-and-that in those conditions?"

If that's what you think, you're a doubter! An unbeliever!

"Oh, I'm not an unbeliever. I love the Lord and I believe the Bible."

Do you believe it all?

"Oh, yes!"

Do you believe in speaking in tongues?

"Well, Brother Norvel, yes, I believe it's for some people, but not necessarily for me."

Well, thank God that you're trying to believe, even though you don't yet. So just keep on and on. The teaching in this Book could help you a lot if you'd let it. Tell God, "Anything that I can read in the New Testament, I'm going to boldly believe it's mine."

And God will say, *Good! Show Me!* And when you start showing Him, He will start manifesting Himself to you. And He will give you anything that you want.

Talk to The Mountains

Jesus tells you how to overcome mountains in Matthew, chapter 21. In this verse, Jesus said, "…if you shall *say* unto this mountain…." You need to talk to mountains. Use your *mouth.*

What's a mountain? "Mountain" could mean a thousand and one things. It could and does mean, for example, disease.

Jesus said to me, *Son, you have to teach the people to talk to the mountains and to the devils. 'Mountains' or problems are caused by devils, so talk to the mountains and the devils and tell them to get out. Pull them out.*

Verse 21 continues, "…if ye shall *say* unto this mountain, Be thou removed, and be thou cast into the sea; it *shall* be done!" Jesus said it! "*It shall be done!*" And it will disappear in the bottom of the sea of forgetfulness. God won't remember that dumb mountain anymore. It will be gone.

In verse 22 Jesus said, "And all things, whatsoever ye shall ask in prayer, believing, ye shall receive." This was the Scripture I used for my text *Confession Brings You Possession* in the small Canadian church.

If you make up your mind to believe God, you will see great things happen all the time. It's amazing what you will see, while the whole church world is sitting around wondering if it's going to happen or not.

To the man in the wheelchair, I said, "Mister, the word of the Lord came unto me saying that what I taught this morning would work for you, *if you would obey it! If* you would obey it!

"I taught *Confession Brings You Possession.* You know, *talk* to your mountains. Look at your crooked legs and call them straight. Talk to them. Tell them what you mean. You can have what you say. Your confession brings possession. Don't say your legs are crooked. Call them straight! Romans 4:17 says that God calls those things which be not as though they were. So, call your crooked legs straight. You do it. Call your crooked legs straight."

He looked at me like he was offended. But I don't pay any attention to offenses when it comes to God's work. That's usually the devil anyhow. I only thought, *God said that confession would bring possession to him, and I'm going to get it into him. I'm going to bombard his mind.*

You see, people's problems are usually with their minds—they don't think straight. I was determined to get this man's thinking straightened out. So I just held on and pulled myself over to him and put my mouth real close to his ear. I said,

"Mister, Jesus said, 'Call your crooked legs straight.'" I repeated this several times. "Call your crooked legs straight."

I guess I said that seventy-five to a hundred times. This old human breath wants to give out, but you have to keep on and not let go. I had to blast this man's goofed up mind away from him. Finally, the man in the wheelchair opened up on the inside and said, "I call my legs straight!"

I said, "Well, thank God for that! Glory to God!" I almost wore myself out for him. You see, some people's minds are so goofed up, you will wear yourself out trying to get the Word of God on the inside of them.

After I got the man in the wheelchair to call his legs straight, I kept encouraging him. "That's right, now you're pleasing the Lord. Keep on saying that."

It was hard for him to get it out, but he kept on. When I had him continually confessing, I backed off. After about five minutes of confessing that his legs were straight, the Spirit of the Lord came and overshadowed him. He *will* do that for *everyone* who *confesses the Bible* and claims it for themselves. He'll do it for you, too!

The man began to cry. And, you know, I had gotten *confession brings you possession* so deep into him, that in the midst of his crying he was still confessing. The Spirit of God was blessing him so much. He kept confessing. "I call my legs straight." I stood there and watched him. He arose from his wheelchair and walked across the front of the church and then walked back.

The pastor said, "He hasn't ever done anything like this before."

I said, "Do you know why? You've never talked *to his crooked legs before.* But *he* talked to them today. He *called them straight,* they became straight, and he received strength from God."

I told his pastor to keep encouraging him. The Holy Spirit gave this man strength because He heard him say the Word. The Holy Spirit listens to you. He listens to every word that you say. And when you start quoting the Bible, the Holy Spirit starts working for you at that moment.

The precious gospel of Jesus Christ doesn't work just for the man in Canada. If *you* will *say* to the mountain, it shall be done for *you!* Jesus said in Matthew 21:21, "If ye have faith, and doubt not...if ye shall say unto this mountain...it shall be done."

Get Rid of Goofed Up Thinking

If you believe that God won't get you out of a wheelchair or that God might not choose to heal you, your thinking is goofed up. You need to have your mind blasted. It's a wonder you even found the church building with that kind of intelligence. Most Christians would believe the Bible a lot more if their dumb heads didn't get them in trouble.

Some people will say, "It sounds good, Brother Norvel. I enjoyed your message, but I'm not going to obey it! I don't have to believe the Lord the same way you do. I have a right to believe my own version of God."

No, you don't. You don't have any rights, you dummy, except to believe Matthew, Mark, Luke, and John just like they're written. You can't dream up a gospel of your own. You don't have any gospel if you have one besides Matthew, Mark, Luke, and John. What you've got is sick! Totally sick!

10

GOD WILL SEND YOU ON MISSIONS FOR HIM

If you don't keep the Word of God before your eyes, then it won't be kept in the midst of your heart. (Prov. 4:21.) When you allow this to happen, then God's Word won't work for you. It absolutely will not! The power of confession has to be released from your mouth, and your mouth will always speak out what's in your heart.

If you have the Word of God in the midst of your heart, and *if you know how to talk,* **God will send you on missions to do things for Him to cause people to live and not die.**

You need to get Luke 9:1 in your heart. If you don't, you might not be able to recognize what God wants you to do. He won't give you a revelation to send you on a mission.

Then he called his twelve disciples together, and gave them power and authority over all devils, and to cure diseases.

Luke 9:1

You have authority over *all* devils and to cure diseases. *You* do! Where do you get the power and the authority? You get it from the Lord Jesus. He gave it to you; you've got it in you, now! But if you don't know this, you'll float along. And being a Christian will never help you. You need to know it so *you* will talk right.

"What do you mean, 'talk right'?"

You have power and authority over all devils, but the power is in the confession part—talking right. Jesus gave you this authority. This Scripture proves it:

> *And these signs shall follow them that believe, In my name shall they cast out devils....*
>
> Mark 16:17

Remember, the devil is always the one who causes harm and damage to human beings.

If I had allowed Luke 9:1 to depart from before my eyes, the Lord wouldn't have sent me on the mission that I'm going to tell you about. And if the sixteenth chapter of Mark which says, "...In my name shall they cast out devils," hadn't been in my heart, I wouldn't have been sent either.

I don't know if God ever does this to you, but it's just wonderful when He comes on me and tells me the very address where I'm to go. He doesn't usually tell me what for; He just tells me to go.

One day I was in a Chattanooga, Tennessee, shopping center. The Lord came on me boldly and told me to go to a certain address. He sent me to a boy whose mind had snapped; there was no one who could help him. He didn't even know his own name. He just sat there in a stupor.

It's important to know God and have God's Word on the inside of you. If you'll study and memorize Scriptures and keep yourself available, God will send you to human beings in need. God sends only people who are available on missions.

You have to know that. You have to *make* yourself available. You need to pray like I do: "Lord, I'm available. Send me where You want to send me. Lord, let my life be a blessing to somebody. *Make my life a blessing.*"

When you study the Scriptures and get them on the inside of you, then you will know how to do something. You will know the power in Jesus' name. You will know you have power and authority *yourself.*

Don't Give Up

I prayed for the boy in Chattanooga, but first I said, "I'll pray for him if everyone else will go out of the room and leave me alone here."

I did that because I had talked to the people and knew that they loved the Lord and were Christians, but they didn't believe right. With a case like this, I couldn't have any unbelief in the room at all or healing wouldn't come.

Jesus did something similar to this when He raised Jairus's daughter from the dead.

And he cometh to the house of the ruler of the synagogue (Jairus),
and seeth the tumult, and them that wept and wailed greatly.

And when he was come in, he saith unto them, Why make ye this ado, and weep? the damsel is not dead, but sleepeth.

*And they laughed him to scorn. But **when he had put them all out....***

...he took the damsel by the hand, and said unto her, Talitha cumi; which is, being interpreted, Damsel, I say unto thee, arise.

And straightway the damsel arose....

Mark 5:38-42

So everyone stayed out of the boy's room and I prayed for him *all night.* When I say I prayed for him, I don't mean I just prayed. At first I prayed for him, *then I confessed* total victory in Jesus' name. I used the power of confession.

I said, "Jesus is stronger than the devil, and in Jesus' name I command this boy's mind to come back to him. Satan, you cannot have this boy. I'm not going to let you have him. I'm not going to turn his mind over to you. The Lord sent me here and I've come to get his mind back for him. In Jesus' name, I command you to *come out of him!* I command you to *let his mind go free!* I command, in Jesus' name, his normal mind to *come back to him!*"

I *said* it! That's the difference between victory and defeat, between knowing and not knowing. Make up your mind to get God's Word before your eyes and into your heart, until you *talk* right. Make up your mind there's victory in Jesus' name and that you'll not accept defeat.

Make up your mind that your confession won't get weak. Remember, once the devil begins to detect a weakness in your confession, he'll keep bombarding you until you're whipped. You'll finally say, "Oh, well," and just walk off.

For eight hours I confessed that boy had a new mind, in Jesus' name. *A new mind!* I wouldn't accept anything else. At four o'clock in the morning I was stronger than I was when I started. This was a *desperate case.* And besides that, it was a case where the Spirit of God specifically directed me to go and *bring victory.* And when God tells you to go to a place and bring victory, you'd better go!

After eight hours of confessing, at four o'clock in the morning, white foam began to bubble up out of his mouth. Saliva began to run out of his mouth and onto the floor. And then his mind began to snap back into him!

Now, I didn't get victory that quickly for my own daughter. A few years later she needed help. Well-known, respected ministers came to talk with her. This one would come and that one would come. But she wouldn't listen to anybody. She kept on with her dope, and I kept on confessing. After three years of prayer and confession, she got victory.

You might say, "That's not the way I do it. I just pray for people one minute, and poof, there it is!" Sure, but I've got news for you—that kind of ministry works for headaches—not for people in mental institutions.

I'd like to take you up to a mental institution, turn you loose, and let you see how much these one-minute prayers work. Yes, they'll laugh right in your face. You have to *break* the power of the devil and *confess* total victory in Jesus' name. You have to stick with it until Satan leaves.

I could take *any* person who was totally possessed of the devil, crippled or anything else, to my home and pray for them *every day,* and God's power would come and make them totally normal. I would wrap myself around them, and put my hands on them in Jesus' name, and talk victory all the time until the miracle manifested. I would stick with it, no matter how long it took. And I guarantee you, God's power would make them normal *every time.*

11

YOU TAKE AUTHORITY
OVER THE DEVIL

God wants you to learn to take authority *over* anything the devil tries to put on you; *over* anything that's not right. Learn to take authority over things that buffet or oppress you from the outside *the very moment you detect them.*

If the devil has come to visit you in the form of disease, *you* can take authority over him (if you're born again by the Spirit of God). *You* can pray and believe for your own healing. Don't put your faith in somebody else; put your faith in the Jesus you read about in the Gospels—Matthew, Mark, Luke, and John— *and be healed.*

Be mindful of the fact that you've got power and authority over the devil. Jesus gave it to us when we got saved:

> *Behold, I give unto you power to head on serpents and scor-*
> *pions, and over all the power of the enemy; and nothing shall by*
> *any means hurt you.*
>
> Luke 10:19

Then he (Jesus) called his twelve disciples together, and gave them power and authority over all devils, and to cure diseases.

Luke 9:1

I'm going to teach you how I stop cancer (or anything else that comes from the devil) dead in its tracks and how you can stop it, too!

"Oh, you mean how *God* stops cancer," you may say.

No, I mean how *you* and *I* stop it in Jesus' name. God doesn't have cancer; He doesn't have any diseases. People get cancers and diseases, and God has given born-again people the power to stop them. It's up to us to tell crippled legs, bad hearts, sick bodies, and empty pocketbooks to straighten out!

Make Up Your Mind To Be a Bible Believer

When Jesus gave His disciples the Great Commission of Mark 16:15-18, He mentioned different signs that would follow the believers. In verse 17, the first sign He spoke of was, "In my name shall they cast out devils." I don't know why that scared people so.

Some pastors say, "I don't know about this. I don't know how to deal with devils. I don't want to get my people mixed up."

Casting out devils is a doctrine of the New Testament church. People who ask, "Why do I have to resist the devil? Why do I have to cast out devils?" are people who've gotten over into their own realm of thinking. They've left the Abraham-kind of faith (see Rom. 4:16-21), and they've left the Jesus-kind of authority.

In 1 Timothy 4:1 the Holy Spirit says:

Now the Spirit speaketh expressly, that in the latter times some shall depart from the faith, giving heed to seducing spirits, and doctrines of devils.

This verse plainly shows that some people will depart from the faith and won't cast out devils like Jesus commissioned. It's a *seducing spirit* that talks you into not having anything to do with casting out devils.

If a devil-possessed person comes to your door and asks you to pray for him, are you ready and willing to say, "Devil, you turn this person loose. I command you in Jesus' name to *come out of him?*" Are you willing to let this be a way of life for you?

It's a part of my lifestyle. I do it all the time, nearly every day. And I know if I don't get the devil out of the person, *it will kill them.* Don't forget, the devil comes to steal, kill, and destroy. (John 10:10.) *You've got to make up your mind that you're going to be a Bible believer!*

If you are a pastor and your congregation has never seen you cast out devils, they're as confused as you are. All some churches have is a confused congregation. They float in on Sunday morning, then they float out being nice. I've got news for you: *Jesus isn't nice to the devil.* And He doesn't want you to be nice to him either. He said to use His name and *throw the devil out of the Church!*

"Are you kidding, Brother Norvel?" you may say. "Every person in the Church is a victor. They're all victors all the time."

That isn't true. There's total victory in the Church only as long as you don't let religious spirits, devils, and your goofed-up friends invade the place. God doesn't want His Church to be invaded by the religious ideas of men. He wants you to stand boldly and throw the devil out. *Take authority over the devil,* cast him out, and get people healed.

Let Jesus Be Like He Is in the Gospels

On my way to Honolulu several months ago, the Lord said to me, *Son, start teaching the Word only. Forget about everything else. Forget it and get it out of your mind. Be free from everything else.* He told me to be free from what my friends or what other church members believed.

Some people have an image of Jesus being like their church service. Realize this: Jesus doesn't go by church services! The services of every church in America are supposed to go by Him.

Jesus is the Head of the Church. Jesus is the Great Shepherd. We're supposed to listen to Jesus and not try to change Him. Jesus, today, is exactly what He is in Matthew, Mark, Luke, and John. He has never changed, and He's not going to change. Oh, God, help us keep our minds under subjection, so that we can leave Jesus alone, and let Him be to us like He is in the Gospels. That's the Jesus we want. He knows how to do *everything!* He has paid the price for *everything!* Know this: Jesus loves us. That means you and me!

If you'll make up your mind once and for all that *the life is in the Word,* you won't have to suffer any longer. The light of God shines down through the Word of God. God doesn't have any shadows. The light is in the Word. What you do with the Word is up to you.

Remember, the Holy Spirit performs God's Word, and the beautiful part of the Holy Spirit is that He performs it for *you!*

He'll perform it *all the time,* for the rest of your life. Anything scriptural that you want, He'll give you.

Learn to put the gospel first and stop putting your own or other people's image of Jesus first.

Quit trying to create your own ideas about Jesus, or listening to your friends' ideas about Him. Always remember this: Jesus is a personal Savior, and *personal* means *you!* And if I can convince you not to change Him, He'll show Himself to you *personally.*

You don't need all of Los Angeles, California, to get God to come to you. *Get alone in your living room and He'll come.* In fact, the Holy Spirit will bring Jesus on the inside of you, just like He is in Matthew, Mark, Luke, and John.

And if you'll accept this, He'll come into your living room and operate on you. He's the best surgeon in the world. He'll come into your living room, stretch your crooked legs out, and make them normal.

And I don't *think* that He'll do it; *I know He will!* He'll free anybody!

Devils Are Where Problems Are

In the New Testament, you're given the right to use Jesus' name to keep *all* devils under your feet. Devils are where you have a lot of problems. The devil himself is a destroyer. He's come to do three things: to steal, kill, and destroy. (John 10:10.) *He's your enemy.*

You and I are in battle. We're trying to get to heaven, but the devil means to stop us. He was thrown out of heaven, and he's mad about it. The devil especially wants to attack human beings because they're created in the image of God, and he's mad at God. (Gen. 1:26.)

The devil wants to turn you into an abnormal creature.

It doesn't matter to him what kind. He wants your body eaten up with cancer. He wants to make you a drunk or a dope addict. He'd like to make you step out on your mate and live with somebody else. The devil doesn't want you to be true to your mate. He doesn't want you to have sex with just your mate—he wants you to have it with two, three, four, or five different people. He'll tell you how good it feels.

Don't Listen to Your Body

Some people walk by their feelings. That will get you into trouble. They say, "But my body wants, my body needs, my body likes...."

Your body lies! You can't live by what your body wants. If you start doing that, you'll stay in trouble.

One day the Lord told me to stop smoking, so I did. That's when I realized how strongly my body controlled my life. I had smoked for twenty years and I didn't see anything wrong with it. At church they had a smoking break between Sunday school and the main service. All my relatives smoked. I thought everyone did. Why should I think it was wrong?

The little children in my church didn't wait until they got big so they could smoke. I used to sneak into a ditch and smoke so no one would see me. I smoked cigarettes, cigars, rabbit tobacco, even corn silks and grapevines. I smoked anything that would burn!

So I said, "Okay, Jesus. I didn't know You wanted me to stop smoking. So if You do, I will, Lord."

I pulled out my cigarettes, slapped them down on the table, and said, "Thank You, Lord. For You, I'll do it."

That was fine, and it sounded nice when I said it; but when you've been used to smoking a pack a day for twenty years, after three or four hours go by, that dumb body of yours will have different ideas.

In a few hours, my jaws began to ache and I heard a little voice talking to me. I knew it wasn't God because it was from my body. My body rose up and said, "I want a cigarette."

I said, "No, you can't have a cigarette." And I mean I wanted one so bad I could taste it. But I said, "No! I've quit smoking!"

It doesn't make any difference to your body what you've decided to do. Your body is only a house that you live in. It's separate, and it has its own goofed up desires.

For example, every time my body sees a coconut cream pie, it wants three pieces—especially when it's homemade coconut cream pie. But I always tell my body, "No, you can't have three pieces, you dummy."

When your body likes something, it says, "I want it, I want it, I want it, I want it!" You have to say, "You desire for pie (or cigarettes or whatever), *go from me!*" I said, "You desire for cigarettes, *come out*, in Jesus' name. *Go from me!*" I had to make the dumb thing leave.

Your body doesn't care what God tells you. It will rise up and demand what it's craving. You have to tell your body to shut up!

I thought I'd put my strong faith to work and make it just fine. But I found out my faith wasn't quite as strong as I thought it was. I had some growing to do.

After eight hours, things got desperate! Walking along, I'd meet people who were smoking. My body would say, "Turn around," hoping that a puff might come through the wind, and I would at least be able to smell it.

I'll never forget the second day. My body was desperate. It started screaming. It didn't stay nice like the first day when it would just say, "I want a cigarette." The second day it screamed, *"I want a cigarette! And I want one right now!"* I would have given a hundred dollars for a cigarette, but I wouldn't let myself have one.

After some tough times, I finally won. But I had to resist my body and its desires, just as I have to resist Satan and his suggestions. I learned that the only way I could gain control over my body was to deny it, to make it serve me rather than for me to be a slave to it.

That's what you must do. You must learn to say "No" to disease just as you say "No" to your body. *But remember, don't go by what your body says.*

When a disease tries to rest in your body, resist the disease and say, "No, disease, I take authority over you, in Jesus' name. *Come out of me!"*

12

You Must Say "No" to the Devil

The greatest word in the world that you'll ever say to the devil is *no*. It's a real short word, but as long as you say *no* to the devil, he can't do anything to you. Even if you're an unsaved sinner and the devil tries to tempt you to commit a sin, say, "No! No! I won't do that." He can't make you do it.

Did you know that the devil can't make you do anything? You have to yield yourself to him.

> *Know ye not, that* **to whom ye yield yourselves servants to obey,** *his servants ye are to whom ye obey, whether of sin unto death, or of obedience unto righteousness?*
>
> Romans 6:16

Always remember: You have to say "yes" to the devil before he can do anything to you. If you start participating with a lying spirit, you will start lying. You have obeyed the devil and the spirit that's tempting you. And you've become what the spirit is.

Watch the company you keep. Be selective about what you let yourself hear, read, or see—on TV for example. The Psalmist David said in Psalm 101:3:

> *I will set no wicked thing before mine eyes: I hate the work of them that turn aside; it shall not cleave to me.*

Good instruction is given in Psalm 1:1, also:

> *Blessed is the man that **walketh not** in the counsel of the ungodly, nor **standeth** in the way of sinners, nor **sitteth** in the seat of the scornful.*

Watch where and with whom you walk, stand, or sit.

You Must Bind the Devil

You must say *no* to the devil. Don't participate with him in any form or fashion. If he has already attacked you, *you must bind him.* Understand this: if the devil has come to you with a disease, bind him first. Then you can effectively resist him.

Concerning the Church, Jesus said, "...the gates of hell shall not prevail against it" (Matt. 16:18). *You have to bind the devil!*

In Matthew 12:29, Jesus said, "...else how can one enter into a strong man's house, and spoil his goods, except he first bind the strong man? and then he will spoil his house." If you want to spoil the devil's efforts, you must first bind him.

Recognize that God *and* the devil exist! The devil isn't dead. As long as you resist evil—like lying, cheating, and diseases—then the devil's hands will be tied and he won't be able to harm you. *But you have to resist him in Jesus' name.*

James 4:7 makes it very clear. "Submit yourselves therefore to God. *Resist the devil,* and he *will* flee from you." Anything that attacks you from the world of darkness—like confusion, heartaches, or pain—is from the devil. Take authority over it *right then,* and in the name of Jesus say, "No, you don't. Not to me you don't, devil, no, no, no!"

Both you and I have power and authority. Any devil I can cast out in Jesus' name, you can, too. Any person I can get healed in Jesus' name, you can, too. *You* can! *God doesn't have any pets or superstars. God has believers!* God doesn't let the gospel work for just a few people; it works for everybody. And if you'll believe the Bible, the Bible will work for you.

If I believe the Bible, it works for me. If I don't believe it, then it doesn't work for me. Because my name is Norvel Hayes and I have authored several books and I have a Bible school, campus ministries, and numerous tape series, that doesn't mean "fifteen cents worth of nothing." The gospel works for everybody and it works the same. I have to say "no" to aches and pains that try to visit my body, "no" to temptation, "no" to the devil just like you do.

Here's how I do it. I say, "In Jesus' name, no, you don't. I won't accept this pain in my side. I bind you, Satan, in Jesus' name. *Go from me!*"

Then I lay my hand on myself and continue, "In Jesus' name, no, I won't accept this. I break your power, Satan, and I command you to take your hands off. My body belongs to God. In Jesus' name, pain, *stop!* In Jesus' name, get off of me. I claim the healing power of God. No, you don't; not to me you don't.

You can't, Satan. I know you want to, but you can't! When I say you can't, you can't!"

How long do I say this? *Until the affliction leaves!*

"But, what if it takes three days, Brother Norvel?" you say.

Big deal! Let it take three days. It probably won't. But if it does, I *keep on*. God doesn't promise that you'll see things happen the very moment you pray. He says:

> ...*What things soever ye desire, when ye pray, believe that ye receive them, and ye shall have them.*
>
> Mark 11:24

When you pray, believe that you receive, and you shall have what things soever you desire. You can have them today, but it may be next week or next month until you have them. But you *shall* have them, if you believe.

Never Change, Never Waver, Never Get Nervous

Once I start resisting the devil, the first morning I wake up the pain may be worse. That's all right—that's a sign I'm getting better.

When you resist the devil, he gets all shook up, and he's going to attack you stronger, because you're resisting him. He means to show us he's stronger than we are, so the next day the pain may be worse.

If it is, I do the same thing I did the first day. *Never change, never waver, never get nervous.* Just lay *your* hand on *your* side, if that's where the pain is, and say, "In Jesus' name, no, you don't. I resist you. I've claimed a healing. The healing power of God is in me *now*. I resist you, Satan, in Jesus' name. Go from me! I command my body to be *free* from you, Satan!"

When you walk back and forth in your own living room, and you do what I've just told you to do, don't let your confession weaken. Do this *every day*, even if it takes four or five days. Your confession must get stronger every day, not weaker. If the devil sees one speck of weakness coming out of you, you've had it! If weakness or doubt comes, he'll dog your tracks right into the hospital. He'll dog you with pain. He'll dog your tracks into the grave, if he possibly can.

The devil doesn't intend to stop or give up. Just show him some weakness and he'll ride you on and on and on. But show him strength and power and you'll stop him!

If you've been binding and resisting the devil and sometimes it hasn't been working, you haven't been doing it right. You haven't been listening to God. You've been listening to yourself. Often, there's a foundation of God that needs to be laid in your life before the victory comes.

James 4:7 first tells you to "submit yourself to God," then it says to "resist the devil, and he will flee." In this book I'm teaching you how to submit yourself to God, so you can get a foundation laid. Then you will be most effective in taking authority over the devil.

It Works Anytime and Anywhere

Taking authority over the devil works all the time and everywhere. You can take God anywhere. He's not nervous.

Once I visited a prison in Lewisburg, Pennsylvania, to counsel with James Hoffa. I also spoke during chapel service. Afterwards I was given fifty-five minutes to talk with the prisoners.

The fellows were lined around the wall, and I was telling them that Jesus is the Alpha and Omega, and that Jesus has everything. They just stared at me. I'm telling you, when you go to places like that, *you'd better know God!* You can be born again and know God pretty well. But, you'd better know Him *real well*—you'd better know what He will and won't do—before you go into prisons.

A great, big bank robber, weighing about 220 pounds, stood up in the crowd and said, "Hey, Mr. Hayes, I'm a bank robber from Washington, D.C. I've got sixteen years in this place. To hear you tell it, it sounds like God will do anything for anybody—even bank robbers."

I said, "That's exactly what I believe. I didn't say God would do anything for you if you don't trust Him. But if I can talk you into trusting Him, I believe God will do anything for you!"

"I've been deaf for thirty years. Would He heal my ears?" he asked me. Then he sat back down.

I said, "Do you want Jesus to heal your ears?"

He said, "I'd like that."

I told him to stand up. When he did, I walked over to him, put my hands on his ears, and said, "You foul deaf spirit, in Jesus' name, *come out of him!*"

The very moment I said that, he fell forward. I caught him in my arms and, boy, was he heavy. By the time I caught him, he was already crying because the Spirit of God had hit him like a lightning bolt. That deaf spirit came out of him.

I stood there holding this guy, while he wept and wept. The other prisoners said, "Whew, God's in this place!"

I said, "You said that right. God came in here in my belly! The kingdom of heaven is *within you*: out of your belly shall flow rivers of living water. (John 7:38.) And it will flow out to *the uttermost.* I've got to go, men. Trust the Lord, and He'll do the same thing for you that He did for this man. Glory to God! Blessed be the name of the Lord!"

The chaplain of the prison came and tapped me on the shoulder and said, "Mr. Hayes, your fifty-five minutes are up and we must go now."

I followed him down a long corridor to the place where I had emptied my pockets (that's a prison regulation).

As we walked, the prisoners came running out of the room where Jesus had opened up the deaf ears of their buddy. They snatched at my clothes. They pulled at me, I mean, really pulled. One little Puerto Rican boy would hardly let me go. He had been given two to three hundred years for shooting and killing a cop. "Mr. Hayes, please come back and help us," he pleaded. "Come back. Please come back and help us. Please come back, Mr. Hayes."

Later I got a letter from the healed man's wife. She told me he could hear perfectly. She thanked me very much for going to the prison and asked me to pray continually for their family.

With all those concrete block walls, prison is a cold-looking place. I used to go to prisons a lot. I love that ministry—a ministry to a world of forgotten men. There's a stigma about a person being in prison that the world isn't sensitive to. But some of the nicest people I've ever met were in prison.

Thank God, we can go into these places and help people get set free by taking authority over the devil. We can do this because Jesus told us that *in His name we can cast out devils!*

13

BE THE HEAD OF
YOUR HOUSE

Whatever happens at my house and on my property *is my fault.* I can't blame the devil, neighbors, or friends. It's my fault. This truth became clear to me years ago when my daughter had over thirty growths on her body.

At that time, I didn't know that God would remove *all* those growths. I didn't know that He would put new skin on my daughter right in my own house. Man didn't teach me about this kind of God with this kind of love and power. *I learned that from no man.* In fact, I don't know very many men who know it and believe it; but *I've found the truth.*

One Sunday night I was praying for my daughter, asking God to heal her of those growths. While I was praying, Jesus came and got me—He pulled me out of my body. I left it there in the living room. I went up into His holy presence. All of a sudden, I was in paradise.

Is that Scripture? If it hadn't been, I wouldn't have gone. It was *His* Scripture. As quickly as you can bat your eyes, God can pull you out of your body and take you to paradise with Him. The Apostle Paul spoke of an experience along this line:

> *I knew a man in Christ above fourteen years ago (whether in the body, I cannot tell, or whether out of the body, I cannot tell: God knoweth,) such an one caught up to the third heaven.*
>
> *And I knew such a man, (whether in the body, or out of the body, I cannot tell: God knoweth;)*
>
> *How he was caught up into paradise, and heard unspeakable words, which it is not lawful for a man to utter.*
>
> 2 Corinthians 12:2-4

After Jesus pulled me out of my body and into His presence, He started talking to me. He looked at me and asked, *How long are you going to put up with the growths on your daughter's body?*

"What do you mean *me*, Lord?" I asked. (Saying something like that doesn't go over very well in heaven!)

He said, You're the head of your house! *Be the head of your house!* (Now I know how the moneychangers must have felt when Jesus ran them out of the temple in Matt. 21:12-13.)

I answered, "*I am!*" This is when I got the inside revelation from God that whatever happened at my house and on my property is my fault.

But how was I supposed to make those growths leave my daughter's body? In the church I came from, I was never taught how to make growths leave.

Jesus said, *You are the head of your house! If you will curse those growths in My name,* they will die! *They will disappear! If you will believe and not doubt, they will die like the fig tree did that I cursed.*

My Daughter Received New Skin

When I came back into my body, I did exactly what the Lord told me to do. For three years I had prayed and those growths were still there. But when Jesus gave me the authority to use His name, and told me what to do and how to do it, I got results!

I went to my daughter and I cursed the roots of those growths on her body. I told them, "In Jesus' name, *you must die!* You're in *my house,* and *you must die!*" After saying this for thirty days nothing happened; in fact, the growths looked worse. But I kept on and on. Finally, after forty days, God's power came into *my* house and swept over my daughter's body.

That afternoon my daughter had come home from high school and walked into her bedroom. All of a sudden, I heard a noise like the dresser falling over. She came running out of her room and down the hallway, screaming, "Daddy, Daddy, this is spooky. This scares me, Daddy. It scares me! Look at me. Look! Look at my legs. Look at my arms. All of the growths are gone! I have new skin on me."

After three years, as quickly as you could bat your eyes, all of the growths disappeared from her body. Jesus put new skin all over her. It looked like baby's skin. *That's the way God does business.*

I don't have to go around wondering what this church believes, or what that church believes. I never wonder whether God will heal club feet, or if He will remove growths and give a person new skin. This is why: If you expect a glass of water from God, He will provide it *for you!* If you expect a healing from God, He will provide it *for you.*

God will do for your child what He did for mine. After forty days and forty nights of believing, it was all over! It was just that quick. All the knots were gone and new skin came on my daughter's body. Jesus came along and replaced the ugly, broken, bleeding places on her hands with new skin.

If you think Jesus won't heal you, you're wrong. He'll do anything for you! He'll do anything scriptural *for you and for your family. Be the head of your house* and pray for yourself and your family. Don't take *no* for an answer.

Your Faith Can Work for Your Children

You can obey the Bible for your children and God will work on their behalf. When they grow up, your faith won't work as well for them. It will only work in part.

Until your children are about sixteen, you can get healings and things for them by using your faith and your confession. But after that, your confession and your faith will only work in part for them.

Eighty-One-Year-Old Woman Gets Healing for Deformed Boy

I remember an eighty-one-year-old woman who was as wild as she could be. It's no wonder she was so wild: she was keeping a blind, crippled, and deformed boy who rolled around and mumbled and groaned. He was living in *her* house and under *her* authority.

She couldn't lift him, so every day she dragged this boy across the floor, saying, "In Jesus' name, *walk!* You're going to walk! In Jesus' name, *walk!*"

And every night she would kneel down by her bed and say, "Oh, Father, in Jesus' name, I pray that You will give this young man a special miracle and a special talent. I want You to give him a special talent."

This went on daily for *three* years. She confessed and prayed. Then one night after she went to bed, she heard someone playing the piano like Liberace. She asked her husband, "Did you hear that? You left the TV on." He told her he didn't think so, but they got out of bed to go check.

What they saw was a young boy sitting at the piano playing better than Liberace. God had come to that deformed boy in the night and made him normal. He had stretched out his deformed limbs and healed them. Then He marched him over to the piano where the boy started playing.

Isn't it wonderful what the Lord did for that boy? He'll do it for your child, too! And you don't need a minister to come and pray to get God to heal your child. Get the religious ideas out of your mind and know that the Scriptures will work for you. Boldly keep the Scriptures in the midst of your heart and let your mouth speak them out. (Prov. 4:21.)

You need to do it yourself. Believe God for yourself. *Be the head of your house!* For three years an eighty-one-year-old woman confessed over a deformed boy, "In Jesus' name, walk! Body, I say unto you, you're in *my house,* straighten out and be normal. Mind, be normal."

Every day for three years she did this, and one night God came and did what she asked. You need to boldly confess the Word of God that covers your case every day. *If you'll say it with victory and with love,* it won't be long, maybe a few weeks, until God will move for you and your family.

You Can Get a Healing
for Your Husband or Your Wife

When you're married, *you can get a healing for your husband or wife* because the two of you are one. God is merciful, and if you obey the Bible for your mate, God will move on their behalf.

Awhile back, a young man was in the hospital unconscious and given up to die. I was the guest speaker at his home church, so they asked me to go to the hospital and pray for him.

His wife was by his bedside. I prayed for him, then I turned to leave. On my way out, the Lord spoke to me and said, *Mark 11:23 would heal him, if it was obeyed.*

When the Lord said that to me, I turned around real quick and went back over to the man's wife. I said, "Young lady, the Lord spoke to me and told me that Mark 11:23 would heal your husband. Now the way to get the Holy Spirit to perform Mark 11:23 is to quote it. It says you can have what you say."

> *For verily I say unto you, That whosoever shall **say** unto this mountain, Be thou removed, and be thou cast into the sea; and shall not doubt in his heart, but shall believe that those things which he **saith** shall come to pass; **he shall have whatsoever he saith.***
>
> Mark 11:23

"Sit here and obey it. Look at your husband straight and say, 'My husband will live and not die, in Jesus' name. My husband will live and not die, in Jesus' name.' Say it strongly all the time.

You may have to say it thousands of times, day in and day out, but don't stop saying it, and he will live and not die."

I got her saying it, then I had to leave. I knew the young man would live and not die, *if his wife kept her confession strong.* Now if she had said it only a hundred times and quit because she got tired of saying it, he would have died. You had better never get tired of talking the Bible if the case is desperate and you want the Holy Spirit to move.

You might say, "Now, Brother Norvel, you don't have to say it so much. You can just believe it by faith."

Why should you mind saying it? Remember, faith has works. (James 2:17.) But I know you can believe God for something and express it once, then thank Him for it. I'm not talking about that. I'm talking about a desperate situation where the Lord told me specifically how to get victory.

Six months later I went back to this young man's area. Before the pastor introduced me to speak, he said, "There's a young man who wants to give a testimony before Brother Norvel teaches tonight."

A Wife Who Refused To Let Her Husband Die

A young man came forward and walked up to the pulpit. He said, "Several months ago I was in the hospital dying. The doctors had told my wife there was no hope. Your speaker tonight, Mr. Norvel Hayes, was holding a meeting here in the church. Our pastor brought him to my room in intensive care. He taught my wife how to confess a verse of Scripture. She sat by my bed and confessed it, and the Holy Spirit healed me."

After he sat down, I asked his wife some questions for the benefit of the congregation concerning his healing. (I wanted to hear her answers, too. I like to hear the way God does things.) I asked her if she kept making the confession I gave her.

She said, "Oh, yes, thousands of times, hours and hours, days and nights. I did exactly what you said."

That's what I call attending to God's Word and not letting it depart from your eyes. (Prov. 4:20-22.) God warns you to do this. Keep His Word in the midst of your heart, and *then* your mouth will confess it. When you confess God's Word, it will be performed by the Holy Spirit.

I asked the wife, "How long did you confess that your husband would live and not die before you saw any improvement? When I left you that day, he wasn't breathing very regularly."

She said she made her confession two hours before there was any improvement in his breathing. After that, it sped up a little bit.

This was a good sign, because for two days and two nights he had only been taking a breath every once in a while. The doctors wouldn't even give him any medicine. They'd say, "Don't get your hopes up. Every breath could be the last. He'll draw one last breath and then stop. And that will be it."

But she kept her confession going, all day and all night. Two days and thousands of confessions later, his breathing returned to normal.

She said, "I said it until I got tired. Then, I'd rest for a minute or two and start again. I said exactly what you told me to say:

'My husband will live and not die. In Jesus' name, my husband will live and not die.'"

Jesus said you can have whatever you say. The power of confession is in *saying* words. Jesus said in Mark 11:23 that you can have, that means "possess" or "own," whatever you say! The young woman said, "*My husband* will live and not die!"

You might say, "I've seen a lot of people like that in hospitals and they died."

No, you haven't either! You've never seen anyone in the hospital die when their wife was sitting by the bed boldly saying, "In Jesus' name, my husband will live and not die," and saying it for days and days without letting up. You've never seen anyone die when somebody paid that kind of price. I'm telling you, the Holy Spirit performs the Bible.

Some people are the nonchalant praying type. They say, "Oh, well, that Mr. Hayes is a nice fellow. But my pastor wouldn't have him at our church. He's a guy who goes around the country saying that you have to confess a lot. I'll just confess a few times and it will probably work." Then when they get tired of confessing, they go get a coke.

That won't work. Have someone bring the cokes to you! Someday your loved one may be dying with no one else to help them except you. Just you! *So pay the price of faith and pay the price of confession* and, I guarantee, you'll see the Holy Spirit work.

In fact, I had this young man's doctor teach at my Bible school a while back. He testified that this young man is the youth leader in his church and totally on fire for God. Thank God for a wife who refused to let her husband die.

14

SHOW GOD YOU TRUST HIM

You have to *show* Jesus that you'll trust Him. There are all kinds of ways you can do this.

One morning many years ago, someone knocked loudly on the door of my home in Cleveland, Tennessee. When I opened the door, there stood a Pentecostal pastor whom I knew very well. At that time I was still a member of the denomination I had been raised in.

He said, "Brother Norvel, I met someone yesterday whom the devil is attacking. It looks like she's dying. Her husband is out of town and her two little children are without food. She can't get out of bed. As I was at the church praying, the Lord spoke to me and said, *Go get Norvel Hayes and let him lay his hands on her and pray for her.* So I came right here to get you."

I was surprised. He was Pentecostal and I thought he knew God better than I did. I asked him *why* he didn't pray for her.

He said, "I did and nothing happened. The Lord told me to come get you and have you lay hands on her. So I came to get you."

I told him I thought he was kidding.

He kept insisting, "No, Brother Norvel, the Lord spoke to me and told me to come and get you. Brother Norvel, she's so bad. She can't get out of the bed and she's aching with pain."

I felt assured that God had really spoken to him. So I agreed to meet him at the church in thirty minutes.

I said, "Honey, that's Jesus healing you! You're being healed this minute. You know it, don't you?"

At the church, the pastor, his song leader, and I got several plates of food for the children and made our way to their house. The dying woman had never been to a Pentecostal church. We walked in, and she was lying in bed moaning in pain. Her precious little children were there, too.

She was a beautiful lady: I thought she was between thirty and thirty-five years old. She said, "Oh, I feel so bad, I can hardly stand it. It hurts so bad."

The pastor was very calm and told his song leader, "You get down at the foot of the bed and pray. I'll get beside the bed."

I didn't know God that well myself, but this pastor did. He said, "Brother Norvel, the Lord Jesus wants you to pray for her, and we'll agree with you."

I walked to the head of the bed and reached out my hand and said, "Now, Satan, you leave this woman alone this minute. In Jesus' name, I command you to take your hands off of her body. Oh, Lord Jesus, Thy healing power, *let it flow.*"

My right arm and hand began to turn warm. And the power of God began to rush through both of my hands. My bones began to ache. The power went into the woman's body, and it began to shake. God's power shook her body and the bed.

She shook real strong for a couple of minutes. Then she said, "What's going into me? There's something going into me that's calming me and the pain is leaving."

I said, "Honey, that's Jesus healing you! You're being healed *this minute*. You know it, don't you?"

She said, "Yes, I am! I'm being healed! All the pain is leaving!" For about two or three minutes, I stood there while the power kept going into her. After that the pain was completely gone and she was totally healed. She stopped shaking and so did the bed.

She took a deep breath and said, "Oh, it's amazing! I'm normal! There's nothing wrong with me. Everything bad has disappeared."

The pastor, the song leader, and I started to walk into the living room. As we were going through the door, I turned around and said, "You're well now. Do you understand that? People who are well are supposed to be up with their house clothes on, walking around and doing their housework."

She said, "Yes, that's right."

Give God the Glory

I closed the door on the way out. As the three of us were getting the food ready for the little children, the woman came walking out, fully dressed. I'd never seen anything like this in all my life. But she walked right by us. You would have thought she would have come out and made an ado over us. But when you learn it's all God, you don't need an ado made over you.

She passed right by us and went over to the sink that was full of dirty dishes. She fixed some dishwater and started washing dishes and singing as she washed. She sang a song to the Lord. As she sang and worked, the joy of the Lord began to boil up out of her supernaturally. She sang and sang and sang. The pastor tried to talk to her, but she kept on singing to God. When we walked out, she was still washing dishes, shouting, rejoicing, and singing at the top of her voice. She was thanking and praising the Lord for her healing.

Make Yourself Dance

"The joy of the Lord is your strength" (Neh. 8:10). I don't have any sad days. I see to it that I don't. The devil is a liar. (John 8:44.) When he tries to give me a sad day, I say, "No, you don't, in Jesus' name. I don't accept this and I bind you. You foul spirit of sadness, *go from me.* You're not going to do anything to me."

Then I start making myself dance. I'll dance before the Lord for two or three minutes. Do I feel like dancing? No! I feel like crying. You have to *make* yourself dance before God. You don't go by feelings: "For we walk by faith, not by sight" (2 Cor. 5:7). David danced before the Lord with all *his* might. (2 Sam. 6:14.)

Make yourself dance for two or three minutes. Then hold up your hands, walk around, and worship God. Worship the Lord, praise Him, and bless the name of Jesus by saying, "I praise You, Jesus. I love You, Lord. I praise You, Jesus."

Sing the Lord a Song

After about three or four minutes of praising the Lord, I sing Him a song. The Word of God highly encourages us to do this.

Sing aloud unto God, our strength: make a joyful noise unto the God of Jacob.

Psalm 81:1

I will sing of the the mercies of the Lord for ever; with my mouth will I make known thy faithfulness to all generations.

Psalm 89:1

O come, let us sing unto the Lord: let us make a joyful noise to the rock of our salvation.

Let us come before his presence with thanksgiving, and make a joyful noise unto him with psalms.

Psalm 95:1,2

O sing unto the Lord a new song; for he hath done marvellous things: his right hand, and his holy arm, have gotten him the victory.

Psalm 98:1

Make a joyful noise unto the Lord, all the earth: make a loud noise, and rejoice, and sing praise.

Psalm 98:4

You may say, "But, Brother Norvel, you can't sing."

Yes, but God likes to hear me! So I sing Him a song because, "The joy of the Lord is my strength!"

Show God you trust Him. Stomp the devil down. Open up your mouth and say, "You're a liar, Satan. And in Jesus' name I bind you!" Don't let the devil give you one fearful thought or painful condition. *Show God you trust Him. Know that you have the victory*—don't just wonder.

15

STICK CLOSE TO THE BLESSINGS

My heart goes out to some people because I know where they are. Jesus knows where they are, too. Many people have never been *taught* what to do to receive from God, or that they even *can* receive from God.

Many have never been *taught* to worship God, to take authority over the devil, or to stand on a verse of Scripture. But it's *all* in the Bible. Jesus told me one day, *Son, always remember this:* people only believe what they have been taught!

In 1 Corinthians 12:2, we read, "Ye know that ye were Gentiles, carried away unto these dumb idols, even as ye were led." *As ye were led,* not as you were forced or driven. You've got to watch whom you let lead or teach you.

Learn To Be at the Right Place at the Right Time

My mother died from cancer at the age of thirty-seven. When I asked Jesus why, I prayed for three days before I got an answer. He told me she died because of the church she went to.

I told Jesus that the church she went to loved Him. But because you love Jesus is no sign that He's going to heal you. You have to be unashamed of Jesus and confess Him daily as your Healer. You have to make Jesus your living Healer, *if* you want Him to heal you.

I have no problems being a good businessman, because I confess Jesus over my business *all the time.* I confess this: "Jesus, You're the best businessman I've ever met. You show me how to invest my money in deals *You* want me to make. I'm not gullible, Jesus. I don't ever have to have another business deal the rest of my life. I'm going to take the Bible and the Holy Ghost and do what You want me to do.

"But, I do confess that You're the best businessman I've ever met. And anytime *You* want me to invest money in something, it will make a good profit at no extra effort. I want that kind of investment. Go before me and get me good investments, ones that I don't even have to work at, because I'm too busy winning souls. Jesus, You're the best businessman I've ever met."

By confessing this way, I make a lot more money than I ever did as a slave to my corporation. And as long as I keep thinking that way, that Jesus is the best businessman I ever met, He becomes that to me. If you confess Jesus as your Healer, He becomes that to you. If you confess Him as your miracle-worker, He becomes that to you. He is to you, *right now,* what you confess Him to be.

Whatever situation you're in, *it's your own fault.* It isn't God's fault, my fault, your friend's fault, or even the devil's. *It's yours! You've been at the wrong place at the wrong time.* You'd better learn to be at the right place at the right time!

When a certain young lady started traveling with me as a singer, she said, "Now, Brother Norvel, I don't want you to give me any money. I'll buy my own plane ticket."

I told her, "Now, honey, I'm going to tell you something right now: If you're going to make that kind of dedication to the ministry of the Lord, the blessings of heaven will fall upon you. And if you dedicate yourself to this ministry and you stay the way you are, the blessings of heaven will fall upon you."

You have to stick close to the blessings. If you don't stick close, you can't get the blessings. They won't be there. Elisha stuck close to Elijah and you see what he got—a double portion of Elijah's anointing. (2 Kings 2.) Proverbs 13:20 says, "He that walketh with wise men shall be wise: but a companion of fools shall be destroyed."

If the man with club feet hadn't stuck close to James 5:14-15, *he wouldn't have gotten new feet.* He had to stick close to the blessing.

God told me once, just as plain as could be, *Son, anybody on earth who loves you and blesses you, I'm going to bless them mightily.* I'm just telling you what the Lord told me. He said, *I'm calling you and I'm anointing you, and I'm going to set you in the office of a teacher.*

Several years ago in Columbus, Ohio, the Lord came right through the wall of my motel room! I had been kneeling beside the bed praying, and it scared me so bad that some of my hair fell out and the meat on my body trembled. I jumped up on the bed and dug my heels into the bedspread. I backed up against the wall like a crayfish. I didn't know that God would put His holiness around you in such a manner that it would scare you.

The Holy Ghost in my belly was jumping and tears were gushing out of my eyes. Then I couldn't see. I thought the meat on my face was going to melt off my bones and go right on the floor.

The Lord started talking to me in a voice. Now I'm not describing some sort of vision that I dreamed up. God Himself spoke to me *in a voice!* And what He told me, of course, has all come to pass. It always does when God says it.

This is what the Lord said, *I've pulled you, son, out of the murky clay. I've cut your feet loose from the net that had you bound. Now I'm going to set you way up on a high hill in this world. And the light of God will shine down to you to many men upon the earth. You must go in peace in Jesus' name.*

After He said, *in Jesus' name,* He disappeared. God had come exactly like the wind and made those statements to me, then He was gone. I was left on the bed trembling and crying, gasping for breath. It took five minutes before I could even see. I said, "Oh, my God, what are You going to do with me?"

The kind of religious training I had received growing up hadn't left me with much sense. However, God let me know that He had some. I still don't claim to have much sense. But God, the One who lives on the inside of me, knows how to do everything. He knows exactly how to save precious souls and heal crippled legs. He knows how to give you a new body. I don't know how. I'm not that smart. But Jesus is. All it takes is the Word of God, and Jesus is the Word. (John 1:14.) Stick close to ministries that aren't ashamed of all that He teaches and represents. If you do, you'll be blessed.

16

STICK CLOSE TO THE GIFTS OF THE SPIRIT

There are several ways a person can be healed. One way is through the gifts of the Spirit: the gifts of healing and the working of miracles, in particular. God has given these gifts to be manifested only as the Spirit wills to the church:

> *Now there are diversities of gifts....*
>
> *But the manifestation of the Spirit is given to every man to profit withal.*
>
> *For to one is given by the Spirit...the gifts of healing....*
>
> *But all these worketh that one and the selfsame Spirit, dividing to every man severally as he will.*
>
> 1 Corinthians 12:4,7-9,11

If you talk about and teach the gifts of the Spirit, the Holy Spirit will manifest the gifts supernaturally, because His Word has been presented.

If you've never talked about the gifts of the Spirit, *you won't be getting very much from heaven.* You need to know that the gifts of the Spirit are the weapons of your warfare. They should be counted as the most precious things in this world to you. Without the gifts, your relationship and experience with God will remain a natural thing. It will be bound to church programs, deacons, hymns, and choir specials. You'll listen to messages preached by Dr. Confused. He's confused, because he goes by man's instructions.

You're just like me, a little human being living on the earth. Even though you have a great power living on the inside of you, you're *never* going to tell God *anything. You aren't the boss of anything.* You're to follow instructions, God's instructions. That's all you're to do. God is the boss and you'd better make Jesus the Lord of your life. You'd better make Jesus the Great Shepherd of all the churches. And you'd better follow *His* instructions, because if you don't, you're in trouble already.

"Trouble?" you may say. "Things are going pretty good, Brother Norvel. I might not be in as much trouble as you think I am."

I'm not talking about just any kind of trouble. The kind I'm talking about is when heaven isn't coming down to your sanctuary and blessing it. Things may be going pretty good in the natural, but souls with twisted legs are coming to your sanctuary and they're leaving the same way. This *isn't* God's will for them.

Jesus loves those precious people. He wants His power to go into them and mold them and give them a miracle. It's available to them. If you're born again, and especially if you've been baptized in the Holy Spirit, *you know it's available for them.* You know Jesus wants to do it! It's not God's will that any man should perish. (2 Pet. 3:9.) It's not God's will that any man should stay sick.

God's will according to 3 John 2 is this: "Beloved, I wish above all things that thou mayest prosper and be in health, even as thy soul prospereth." And according to Acts 10:38, "Jesus...went about doing good, and *healing all* that were oppressed of the devil; for God was with him."

Go Where They Teach the Gifts

I have a Southern Baptist friend down in Baton Rouge, Louisiana, who began to teach on the gifts of the Spirit. And he prayed for the sick, too. He had a missionary conference of 2,500 people and invited me to come and speak. I usually go to his church about once or twice a year. It's one of my favorite places in the whole world because he's such a precious pastor.

One night, while I was speaking, some people stood up about halfway back in the large sanctuary. I said, "What's going on back there?"

They said, "A crippled girl stood up!"

I said, "Blessed be His holy name! Jesus likes for crippled girls to stand up. Just tell her to come up here. Come on, little darling." She came walking down the aisle. She looked like she was about fourteen years old. The fellow walking beside her looked about sixteen.

The young boy walking beside her said, "This is my crippled sister. I helped her get in here. I take her everywhere. Oh, God, I helped her get in here."

She was crying as she walked forward, just as normal as anybody else would walk. Her brother could hardly believe it! By the time he got down front, *everybody* knew she *used to be* his crippled sister.

I asked the little girl to tell the people what happened. She said, "I don't know! I was just sitting there with my brother, listening while you were teaching. All of a sudden my legs began to turn warm. After they had turned warm for a few seconds, they began to turn hot. And I felt some kind of strength come into them. I reached down and pushed myself up. *I stood up.* And when I did, both of my legs went completely normal!" Blessed be God forever!

This healing illustrates the gift of the working of miracles. It's a gift to the church. You don't have to pray for it. The gifts are all free for you! All you have to do is believe, and the Holy Ghost will come and do it!

You may think that the Spirit of God *always* manifests Himself to agree with *you and your church.* No. He doesn't agree with you or your church. He agrees with Matthew, Mark, Luke, and John. He agrees with the rest of the New Testament. He agrees with all of God's Word. The Holy Ghost can't stand ignorance! He hates it because it keeps Him from manifesting Himself to you. We are told in Hosea 4:6, "My people (God's people) are destroyed *for lack of knowledge....*"

"Don't you think, Brother Norvel, that somewhere in the world, there might be a case where it's not the Lord's will to heal?"

No! And neither does God! First Corinthians 12:7 says, "But the manifestation of the Spirit is given to *every man* to profit." It doesn't say, "Every man, *except you.*" *Every man* means *you.*

Jesus wants to heal *you* right away. He can hardly wait for me to finish this teaching so He can heal you. That's how bad He wants to do it.

So far I've taught you that Jesus heals you through your own faith in the Bible. By the authority of God, the Lord has given you power over devils and diseases. This requires *you* to pray for yourself and walk the floor every day, boldly saying, "No, you don't, Satan. You're not doing that to me. I won't accept this disease, in Jesus' name. *No, you don't!* Jesus is my Healer!"

The second way I've taught you that Jesus heals is through the gifts of the Spirit—particularly the gift of the working of miracles and the gifts of healing. Now, remember, the gifts of healing (along with the other gifts of the Spirit) operate as the Spirit wills. (1 Cor. 12:11.) *But you need to go to the right kind of church!* The more the pastor teaches and preaches on the gifts, the more they will come into manifestation.

God Will Perform Surgery on You Through the Gifts

Not very long ago I was speaking at a large Bible school on the gifts of the Spirit. The place was packed full of people. I had been speaking awhile when the word of the Lord came unto me saying, "I'm healing right now."

I shouted, "Glory to God! Jesus said He's healing somebody right now!" At that moment, a woman sitting in the audience broke down and began to weep *as the Lord healed her!*

I told the congregation to watch the healing power of Jesus. It flowed, and we all watched it. Then, the Lord began to heal people all over the auditorium. I walked the floor and praised God, showing *great* patience.

You've got to have patience to get God to do very much. If you don't have patience, God will let you do it. And if you do it, you'll get nothing but a little bit of blessing. There won't be a great miracle from Him like receiving an operation. You can receive surgery *today!* Jesus will operate on you if you'll just trust Him. He'll make you a new heart. *But He performs miracles like operating on people in churches where they aren't ashamed to teach and preach about the gifts of the Spirit.*

Sometimes God will move upon me when I'm out teaching, and He'll say, *Son, let Me out there tonight. I want to operate tonight! I want to perform surgery.* He doesn't do this very often. Most people can't stand it, and most churches aren't ready for it. Why? Because they don't teach it or preach it. If you're ever in a service where God operates, I'll guarantee you that you'll never be the same.

When God wants to perform surgery, it must be very quiet and reverent like the Holy of Holies. When God operates, He gives new ribs, new hearts, new feet, and brand-new eyes.

The Lord likes things a certain way when He manifests like this. Several years ago He told me, *Now, I won't perform surgery if someone is playing the piano. I won't perform surgery if people get up and walk around. I won't perform surgery if any kind of instrument is played. I won't do it! I either get the glory or I don't get it!*

He'll give you anything you want. But you'll never get it through nonchalant flaking off and doing what you want to do. God will do anything for you that's scriptural if you'll believe and give Him the glory.

Sometimes He'll lay people out on the floor for two hours and operate. He cuts out cancers and gives them everything new in their body. It's so holy you can hardly stand it. All you really want to do is get on your face before God and just lie there.

The average church in America doesn't even know that God wants to do things like this. Why, God will operate on you while you read this book. Jesus has come to give you what you need. Jesus loves His Church, He loves His people, and He *always* wants to come and heal them—*always.*

His heart and His compassion go out to you when you're sick, or when you're lost, or when you have a broken heart. I can't do much for you except give you some instruction, but Jesus can give you anything you want. Not only *can* He give you anything you want—He's here *now* to give it to you. All He requires of you is for you to reach up to Him like a little child and begin to say, "Jesus, I believe. I believe, Jesus!"

Jesus loves His Church. He's dealt with me about that for years. He said, *Son, the* power *is* in the Church. *I gave My power over to the Church, and they have My name. That's where the power is. The name is where the power is.*

Jesus said, "Hitherto have ye asked nothing in my name: ask, and ye shall receive, that your joy may be full" (John 16:24).

Let the Lord hear you today. Let the Lord fix your heart *now.* If you're on dope, hold your hands up to Jesus and let Him come. He will wipe that addiction away from you this moment, and you'll *never* have to go through cold turkey. Not for one moment. Jesus will set you free from the craving *right now.* He will dry it up!

Are you desperate, and does it seem that nobody in the world loves you? Do you have a sick body, and you don't know where to go for help? Do the doctors say there's no hope for you? I've got news for you: the greatest physician in the world is here right now. He doesn't use any instruments, and He won't be cutting on you. But He will impart to you what you want and need, and remove from you what you don't want or need.

Let the Spirit of God set you free. Men don't have any power to help you. The Holy Spirit can and will do everything that needs to be done. Receive from God now. Oh, the holiness, compassion, and understanding of God bypass all natural understanding! Glory to God!

Many times the Lord wants to move and perform surgery. Seek Him and He'll talk to you about it. And if you're a pastor, tell Him your church is open for this movement of His Spirit. Evangelists, tell Him that *your* ministry is open for it! Speaking and teaching the Bible is wonderful, but when the Holy Spirit wants to do something, *let Him do it—don't fight it.* If you'll do this, you'll see great and mighty things happen. Stick close to the ministries that teach and preach that God moves like this. *Then let Him do it!*

17

STICK CLOSE TO THE LAYING ON OF HANDS

Another way to receive healing is through the laying on of hands. In my opinion, this is the lowest form of faith. The highest type of faith receives healing by believing God's Word on your own. The gifts of healing, which are supernatural manifestations of God, heal any affliction. They manifest when they are taught and preached.

The laying on of hands is God's way to heal so that nobody is left out. And that means *you*. It's a doctrine of the Church. The last words that Jesus spoke before He went to heaven are found in the sixteenth chapter of Mark: "...they shall lay hands on the sick, and they shall recover" (v 18).

In another portion of Scripture in the book of Acts, Jesus is instructing Ananias to go lay hands on Saul of Tarsus that he might receive his sight.

And there was a certain disciple of Damascus, named Ananias; and to him said the lard in a vision, Ananias. And he said, Behold, I am here, Lord.

And the Lord said unto him, Arise, and go into the street which is called Straight, and inquire in the house of Judas for one called Saul, of Tarsus: for, behold, he prayeth,

And hath seen in a vision a man named Ananias coming inn and **putting his hand on him,** *that he might receive his sight.*

Then Ananias answered, Lord, I have heard by many of this man, how much evil he hath done to thy saints at Jerusalem;

And here he hath authority from the chief priests to bind all that call on thy name.

Acts 9:10-14

Sometimes people make fun of healing services with the laying on of hands. They're really making fun of things Jesus told the Church to do in His name.

The story continues:

But the Lord said unto him (Ananias), Go thy way: for he is a chosen vessel unto me, to bear my name before the Gentiles, and kings, and the children of Israel:

For I will spew him how great things he must suffer for my name's sake.

And Ananias went his way, and entered into the house; and **putting his hands on him** *said, Brother Saul, the Lord, even Jesus, that appeared unto thee in the way as thou camest, hath sent me, that thou mightest receive thy sight, and be filled with the Holy Ghost.*

And immediately there fell from his eyes as it had been scales: and he received sight forthwith, and arose, and was baptized.

Acts 9:15-18

Thank God for the ministry of the laying on of hands. Blessed be the name of the Lord!

One night I was at the altar praying for people. I was watching how the pastor did it, because where I came from, we didn't lay hands on anything. We just shook hands and stayed nice. You can't get healed by shaking hands and staying nice.

On this particular night, the healing power of God came into my hands for the first time. It felt like the bones were going to jump right out of my fingers. They tingled and tickled.

I walked over to the full gospel pastor and said, "Pastor, something is in my hands, and it feels like the bones are going to jump right out of my skin. What's this in my hands?"

He told me it was the healing power of God. I was amazed. He brought me over to a dear sister who had been sick for a long time, and he told me to lay hands on her.

I laid my hands on her in Jesus' name and she fell on the floor. I said, "Oh, my God, I hurt her."

The pastor said, "No, that's the healing power of the Lord, Norvel."

Well, I never dreamed that the healing power of the Lord would ever flow through my hands. But it did, and it still does. Since that night, I've seen many more healings as the result of the laying on of hands.

Who Do You Say Jesus Is?

One Sunday morning I was in Pensacola, Florida, preaching to about a thousand people. I was building up the Lord and firing away from Matthew, chapter sixteen. As I spoke about the power of Jesus being turned over to the Church (vv. 18,19), I heard these words on the inside of me, "Who do you say that I am?" You need to ask yourself the question: *"Who do I say Jesus is?"*

Can you *say* without shame that Jesus is a Healer? Would you run a big ad in your hometown newspaper that said, "We're going to have a healing service on Sunday night. Bring all of the sick and demon possessed"?

If you're ashamed of Jesus and His healing power, He will never come into your church and heal crippled people. Not one! You'll push their wheelchairs in for twenty-five years, then push them out, and the people will die like that. And it will be *your* fault. It's not the Lord's fault, and it's not the Bible's fault. Jesus is the Savior; Jesus is the Healer. Jesus is the best surgeon there is. Who do *you* say Jesus is? (Matt. 16:15.)

Total Cripple Walks Off

I was preaching hard that Sunday morning, really pounding away on Matthew sixteen. Power filled the place while I was preaching. And the Lord told me to go lay hands on a twisted, crippled lady sitting in a wheelchair in the audience. I found out later she was almost completely blind, too. I went and touched her on the forehead. When I did, the Holy Spirit's power picked her body up out of the wheelchair and floated her through the air.

This happened in front of about one thousand people on a Sunday morning. The Holy Spirit whirled her right through the air, and when she hit the floor everything about her was normal: her hands, her feet, her eyes. (Today she walks in high heels.)

That Sunday afternoon, she pushed her wheelchair back to the nursing home where she was staying. The people stared at her; some of them fell on the floor and gave their lives to God. Some of those who looked at her body—which was healed from head to toe—fell on the floor and asked God to heal them, too.

That afternoon she sat on the side of her bed and moved the bars out of her way. For years, bars had been around her bed to keep her from falling out. All afternoon the nursing home people came into her room and looked at her.

They were amazed at what God had done. In a split second, she had gone from a blind, twisted, and deformed invalid into a normal woman. This woman had never had any earthly idea that God even did things like this. But He did and still does. He makes the crippled to walk and the blind to see.

Jesus heals *all* diseases. Nothing is too great for Him. Jesus said "...all things are possible to him that believeth" (Mark 9:23). All He wants are believers. So believe! And stick close to the blessings!

18
PUT THE GOSPEL FIRST

Once while I was sitting around at my mission in Florida, the Lord told me, *This coming Easter I want you to go to Fort Lauderdale and pass out tracts to the college students. There will be thousands of students there who are lost and going to hell, and I want you to pass out tracts.*

I had planned to buy a new suit and go to church with my relatives on Sunday morning. Then we were going to go out to dinner and would probably sit around and talk for hours. I hadn't seen my relatives for a long time.

But when God told me to go to Fort Lauderdale, Florida, on Easter and pass out tracts, I just said, "Lord, I'll go! I'm available. Glory to God!" This may shock you, but God doesn't have any big shots. All God wants are human beings who will take orders.

Make Yourself Available to God

"Brother Norvel, if I had four Cadillac cars, eleven businesses, a live-in maid, three homes, three condominiums, and enough money to last the rest of my life, I'd be beyond passing out tracts in Florida. Do you understand that?"

Yes, I understand that's the way most Christians are. And that's the reason many of them get in trouble, because they won't obey God. I didn't say that Jesus told you to go to Florida and pass out tracts or do something else. You might not be available.

Jesus usually tells you to do only things that you're available to do. You have to *make yourself available*. And you have to make yourself available *for anything*. Then Jesus will give you missions to go on to get people set *free!* I just love for God to give me little things to do. When I pray, I ask God to send me anywhere He wants me to go. You'd be surprised to what extremes God goes just to have me bring a blessing to someone.

Obey God. But don't get under condemnation and do things just because Brother Norvel told you to. I'm not leading you; the Holy Spirit is leading you. Those who are led by the Spirit of God, they are the sons of God. (Rom. 8:14.) Make yourself available to God for anything that He wants you to do and be *willing* to do it. Then God will come and deal with you personally and tell you exactly what to do.

The Holy Spirit may wake you up at six o'clock in the morning and tell you to go tell people about Jesus on the city block four streets down. What will your reaction be? Will you say, "I'm not going to do it. I kind of feel like I should, but I just don't want to"? If that's your reaction, the Holy Ghost will say, *If you won't go for me, that's okay.*

Jesus will give you a few more chances. He'll say, *I want you to do this for Me over here. Would you go over and do this for Me?*

Would you answer, "No, I won't do that"?

I went to Fort Lauderdale and passed out tracts all week long. I thought I would be the only one there obeying God, but I found out that God has other people besides me.

Jesus had sent young Christian boys and girls from all over the country to pass out tracts. Many of them recognized me and said, "Oh, Brother Norvel, what are you doing down here?" I told them I was passing out tracts, too. They begged me to teach them.

Since I was going to be there all week, I had lots of time. So I went over to the Garden Building, where they had a room that would seat a hundred people, and I spoke there at night. During those nights, the anointing of God would come upon me stronger, I believe, than ever before in my life.

During the day, these Christian young people would go out on the beaches and bring in those who were strung out on dope and just about ready to go over the edge. They thought their dope was really cool stuff.

I instructed my go-getters to reach out and love those beach kids and tell them the truth. All you have to do is just preach the gospel. If you would learn this, you could get God to do a lot of things for you. Always tell people what Jesus can do for them and how much He loves them.

I would say to those kids, "The Lord is the best heart surgeon there is. He's the best physician I've ever met. I'm telling you, He has the love, power, and compassion to drive out all craving for dope and *make you free!*"

When you're teaching like that, God will come in and knock people out on the floor. You'll watch each one fall like a sack of potatoes. And that's just what happened. I stood up there being nice and told the Holy Ghost, "Get 'em!"

You might say, "Brother Norvel, you sure have an unusual way of spreading the gospel."

I know it, but it works! I've never been to seminary or any Bible school; I just let the Holy Ghost tell me what to do. The Holy Ghost told me He wanted to train me, and He did. That's the reason I'm so wild, because sometimes the Holy Ghost is wild! He'll do anything to help and bless people.

Be Willing To Bring Blessings to Others

It's amazing where the Holy Ghost will send you to bring blessings to people. God doesn't want you beaten down by dope. He doesn't want you walking down the highway with no place to sleep and no food to eat. Let me share with you what He can and will do in a case like this.

One time I was planning to go to the Kansas City Full Gospel Business Men's Convention. I was supposed to leave on Wednesday. But the Lord spoke to me and said, *Don't go to the convention in Kansas City tomorrow. I don't want you to go. I want you to go to the prayer meeting tomorrow night at a little Pentecostal church.*

I knew the pastor very well. We had shared many experiences in God.

I said, "Lord, I want to go to the Kansas City Full Gospel Business Men's Convention tomorrow."

The Lord said, *Don't go! I want you to go to the prayer meeting.*

What would you have said? Some people would say, "I've already made my reservations. I'm not going to that prayer meeting. I'm going to the convention."

The Lord might have responded, *Well, okay. You can go on if you want to.* And He might ask you to do something four or five more times. But if you keep insisting on doing your own thing every time, finally, *He won't bother you anymore.*

If that's happened with you, God probably hasn't come to you with an assignment in years. Why? Because *you do your own thing.* If you're not going to obey God, why would He want to fool with asking you to do things for Him? God is looking for people who will *obey* Him.

I had no earthly idea why God wanted me to go to the prayer meeting at the little Pentecostal church when I wanted to go to Kansas City, but I obeyed and went. That night after the pastor preached, he gave an invitation. One woman came forward out of the small crowd. (Only small crowds show up on Wednesday nights in a lot of churches.)

The woman went down and got on her knees before God. I had never seen her before; but after the prayer, the Spirit of God came upon me and I broke and began to weep. The Lord spoke to me and said, *I want you to give that woman $100 and the table and chairs in your house.*

Weeping and crying, I grabbed my checkbook out of my pocket. God was blessing me so much that I could hardly see the checkbook. I was trying to write, but I had to keep wiping my eyes so I could even see.

The Lord told me to give the check to the pastor, and to tell him that I was to give my table and chairs to this woman.

Double-Mindedness Can Be Dangerous

I walked up to the pastor and gave him the check. As I wept, I told him what God had said. I asked the pastor to please send a truck to my house after the service to pick up the furniture. I didn't want to wait until the next day *because I knew it was the right thing to do, and I didn't want time to change my mind.* Double-mindedness will cause you to miss out on the will of God.

If I had gone to the Kansas City Convention, the Lord wouldn't have turned against me. He loves me, and He loves you. I could have gone, had a good time, and enjoyed the speakers. But that wouldn't have been God's *perfect* will—it would have been His *permissive* will. God's perfect will was for me to go to the little prayer meeting because the Spirit of God told me to.

The pastor told his congregation, "Many of you don't know this woman. I was driving down the road today and saw her walking with her two little children. I stopped, introduced myself, and asked her where she was going. She said, 'I don't know.'

" 'I'm from Germany, and I married an American soldier. We have two children, and he left me. I'm having to raise the children by myself. I was living in somebody else's apartment and using their furniture, but I had to move out this morning. My children and I started walking down the highway. We have no food or money and nowhere to go.'"

The pastor told her he would get her and the children a motel room for the night. He told her he wanted her to come to church with him.

"Every time God sends Brother Norvel Hayes here something good happens. The Spirit of God has dealt with Brother Norvel to give this woman his table and chairs and $100. We had better obey God. All of you who want to help this woman, bring her a gift."

They all began to come down to the front and bring her gifts. Someone gave her a couch. Another one gave her a bed. Someone else gave her a stove. Another person gave her a refrigerator.

Jesus knew this woman was going to be at church that night, and He knew that I would obey Him. That's the reason He wanted me to go to the service.

Ten days later the pastor came by my office and took me to a house where the woman now lived. He told me it was all paid for and full of furniture. He said the woman wanted me to pray for her to get a job. She spoke in broken English and nobody wanted to hire her.

I told the pastor, "Sure, I'll pray for her. *And* God will give her a job." I tell people all the time that if I pray for them, they're going to receive!

You've got to be available, or you will never get the blessing. I don't know what kind of a blessing you'll get or when you'll get it. God refuses to tell human beings a lot of things, but I can tell you one thing: on down the highway of life, maybe even several years later, because you obey Him in what He says to do, God will give you something big like a condominium on the beach.

Put the gospel first. Don't ever pray about whether you should read the Bible! Don't ever pray about going to church or knocking on doors! The Bible is always true, before you pray and after you pray.

Don't ever pray about whether you should go out winning souls, or about having soul-winning revivals, because when you do, you open the door for the devil to come in and talk to your mind. And he will say, *Well, you can wait until next month before you have a revival. Don't do it now. Wait.*

Anytime you want to win souls, don't even pray about it, just go do it. Anytime you want to knock on doors and pass out tracts, just get up out of your seat and go do it.

Your Pride Will Rob You

Some people may say, "Knocking on doors isn't my ministry."

When I hear people say that, I always ask, "Do you have chapter and verse for that?"

"No," they say. "But I don't feel like it's my ministry."

You don't feel like it's your ministry because of your dumb pride. Your pride will rob you of the blessings of God! Get rid of it!

I can see why some might say that knocking on doors isn't their ministry because they might get yelled at. You might knock on a door, then tell the person who opens it, "I want to pray for you and talk to you about Jesus."

They might react like this: "Jesus! I don't even believe in Him; and besides that, they ought to put people like you in jail for invading people's privacy." Then they slam the door in your face.

I guarantee that when that happens to you, the devil will come in like a flood and say to you loud and strong, *This is not your ministry.* You'll think it's God talking to you.

As you're standing there with your pride all bruised, like a sheep-sheared dog, you will agree with him. You'll say, "Yes. Where's my car? I'm going to go back to my church where they're nice."

Yes, it's good to go to church where they're nice; but *the world is going to hell!* That's why you must be open to witness for the Lord anywhere.

God Is Counting on Us

I have a mission in Crystal River, Florida. It's a little mission where we knock on doors to win elderly people to Jesus. One day a guy came walking into my mission and a woman there asked him, "Do you know Jesus?"

He said, "Oh, yes. I'm a Christian because I was born in Crystal River." He didn't know he had to be born again by the Spirit of God.

Some people have let the devil sell them a bill of goods. It's amazing the number of people who think they're Christians because they were born in America. God is counting on you and me to reach these people, to help them live and not die. God is counting on us to make ourselves available to the gospel, to seek first the Kingdom of God.

19

FACE TO FACE WITH TOTAL VICTORY

I have a friend who has a good-sized business. One day he told me that one of his secretaries had cancer.

He said, "She's eaten up with cancer and has been operated on twice. She's lost weight until she's just skin and bones and all of her hair has fallen out. The doctors say she's so far gone they can't help her. They sent her home to die." Then my friend asked me, "Does she have to die?"

I told him, "No, God will heal her." He asked if I would minister to her. I told him, "Sure." So he called her. That night she came over to his home. I took my Bible and went into the living room to talk to her.

I said, "Now, honey, it's my understanding that you know your surgeons have sent you home to die. I probably wouldn't have mentioned it otherwise, unless the Lord led me."

"Yes, they've sent me home to die," she told me. "'No hope for you,' is what they said."

Now pay close attention to what I told her. One of these days, by and by, when the devil tries to destroy you, you'll need to know this. And remember, the devil *always* comes. Nobody is too spiritual for him to try and attack. However, the outcome of his attack will depend on what you do.

I told this secretary, "You don't have to die! Get that straight! *You can live and not die!* But unless you do what Jesus said to do, you *will* die."

The doctors weren't crazy. They were telling the woman the truth. From the natural standpoint, if she left the cancer alone she would die. But, if she obeyed the instructions of the Lord, she could live. I don't care what church you go to, if you accept the doctor's diagnosis and leave cancer alone, it will kill you.

I told my friend's secretary, "I'm going to teach you what Jesus says. You are born again, right?"

"Oh, yes!" she said.

"Now, I'm just an instructor—I don't have any power apart from God. But I'm going to teach you how to live." This will work for you, too.

Here's what I told her: Jesus said in Matthew 21:21 to talk to the mountain. (And that's the way you have to do things—not your way, but God's way.) Now "mountain" means problem. In her case, it was cancer. According to verse 21, first you must have faith and doubt not. Then "...if ye shall say unto this mountain, Be thou removed, and be thou cast into the sea; it shall be done."

Obeying the Scripture I said, "In the name of Jesus, I'm going to curse that cancer. In Jesus' name, I'm going to command it to stop tonight. Right where it's at, it's going to stop, now!"

Notice I didn't say I was going to heal her. I said, "In Jesus' name, I claim my rights and I'm going to stop it."

The reason I can do this is because it's Bible. Jesus is the Healer, but He told us, "...Whatsoever ye shall bind on earth shall be bound in heaven..." (Matt. 18:18). *You* bind on earth, and it's done in heaven. That's *why* you can bind cancer and stop it in its tracks.

Understand this: it's the Spirit of God who does the work. And you get Him to do the work because you claim the written Word of God, in Jesus' name.

If you're dying like this woman was, how can you get the Holy Spirit to work for you? First of all, either you (yes, you can!) or someone else, bind the disease and say, "No, you can't kill or destroy this person (or me) in Jesus' name."

Remember this: when you *say*, "No, you can't," then the devil can't. I'm telling you, he can't!

Face facts. Just like I told my friend's dying secretary: You're going to have some responsibility in getting healed or getting any mountain out of your life. This is where your *mouth* comes in and begins to work. Jesus said, "...if ye shall say unto this mountain." You're going to have to talk to it. Stop dreaming about it. Dreaming doesn't work.

Keep Your Confession Strong

Now open up your understanding to God's Word. Get *every* word. You can't listen to part of what Jesus says then do your own thing. If you'll listen to what Jesus is saying to you, you can receive *whatever you* want from God. Jesus doesn't stutter. His Word is plain. His words are for your benefit to give you *perfect* instructions on *how to receive*. You *receive* by talking to mountains. This is what Jesus said.

When I first taught this sick, dying woman to confess her healing, she would confess a little weakly, "Cancer, you can't kill me."

I said, "Honey, that won't work. Say it *strong*." When the Apostle Paul was administering healing to the cripple at Lystra, Paul said, *with* a loud *voice*, "...Stand upright on thy feet..." (Acts 14:10).

You may have to walk the floor *every day,* saying *loudly,* "In Jesus' name, cancer (or whatever other mountain there is in your life), you'll never kill me. I'm talking to you, and I'm telling you now, get out of my body, my life. Disappear now! Get totally out! You'll have no part of me because Jesus is my Healer."

Jesus Becomes What You Say He Is

Remember you have to *confess* Jesus as your Healer. And don't let the devil talk you out of it! Always confess it *boldly,* and He will become your Healer. That's what Jesus always does— every day of your life—*Jesus* becomes to you what you say He is.

He's the Alpha and the Omega, the beginning and the end. (Rev. 1:8.) He's like that from the beginning until you draw your last breath. *If* you will confess Him as victory in your life, He becomes that to you.

Jesus is your Savior. He's your *Healer.* He's your *miracle-worker,* your *surgeon,* your *love-giver.* He's everything *good* to you. He's the beginning and the end of your life. He's paid the price for *everything* you ought to receive. Understand that He becomes everything to you that you confess and believe the *moment* you say it!

Keep this in your heart. Jesus watches your faith. Remember what He said: "…If ye have faith, and doubt not…if ye say unto this mountain, Be thou removed…it shall be done" (Matt. 21:21). It *shall* be done all the time.

I worked and taught the secretary all these things that I've written here. Like a broken record, I went over it again and again. I had to make sure she got it. I told her, "I'm not going to let you die, honey. You're too willing to die, and there's no use in it. So just give me your hand, and let's walk and confess."

We confessed and confessed. I made her promise me that she would do what Jesus *said.* I warned her, "If you don't do what Jesus said, you're going to die. Do you understand?"

She said, "I understand." And she confessed and confessed.

She Lived!

The Lord created meat on those long, bony arms! God manifested cancer-curing power in her, and she lived!

Later the lady testified at one of my meetings. After I told the congregation basically what had happened, she came forward. The congregation went wild with rejoicing.

A totally healed woman walked on stage. Her body that had been skin and bones now had meat on it. Her bald head was now full of hair. A human being that had been beaten down by the devil and given up to die was alive! This woman is a testimony to the glory of God!

She said that she followed what I taught her. *Every day,* almost twenty-four hours a day, over and over, she told cancer it would be uprooted and removed to the very seed according to what Mark 11:23 says. She read the Gospels again and again. She wrote down all the Scriptures that pertained to healing.

She clung to God's Word confessing that it was sure and that it would stand forever. (Isa. 40:8.) All this time, she was a mess. And the devil would hound her all the time, saying, "You're a dying lady, scrawny and bald."

But do you know what she told him? "Devil, *Jesus* has come to give me life and life more abundantly according to John 10:10. According to 1 Peter 2:24, Jesus took my infirmities and bore my diseases!"

You can live and not die! The Lord, the Holy Ghost, will manifest what you say. Confess Jesus as your Healer *every day.* Confess that disease can't kill you.

Every day walk the floor confessing victory and that the Holy Spirit will begin manifesting Himself. He has all kinds of power and all kinds of personalities. Whatever power you need to overcome your mountain, He will deliver that to you.

Devils Get Nervous

Devils hate me because I won't let them snuff people's lives out. I take Jesus and the Word of God and rescue them. A lot of times when I'm ministering to people, the devils rear up. They scream, they fall on the floor, often they look at me and say, "I hate you." Things like that happen all the time. It's like drinking a glass of water. After a while, you don't pay any attention to it.

A well-known minister's son asked his dad once, "Daddy, Brother Norvel and I were at a meeting in Illinois when suddenly a young fellow rose up and began to scream. That's happened before, too. People would rise up, scream, and throw a fit. Why does that happen in his meetings?"

His dad told him I was a threat to the devils in those people. The devils know it, and it makes them nervous.

If you're dying from some disease right now, the spirit that caused you to get that way is a nervous wreck because you're reading this book! Do you know why? *You're about to come face to face with total victory!* Glory be to God forevermore!

20

JESUS WANTS TO
HEAL YOU NOW

Jesus loves you and wants to heal you *now*. But more important to Jesus than your healing is the condition of your soul. *This must come first.*

> *For what shall it profit a man, if he shall gain the whole world, and lose his own soul?*
>
> Mark 8:36

> *...for it is profitable for thee that one of thy members should perish, and not that thy whole body should be cast into hell.*
>
> Matthew 5:30

The fact of the matter is that Jesus wants your members (body) to be whole *and* for *you* to go to heaven, too. But, you must be born again. (John 3:5.) Your soul comes first and your healing is second. John says it like this:

> *Beloved, I wish above all things that thou mayest prosper and be in health, even as thy soul prospereth.*
>
> 3 John 2

Be in health *even as thy soul prospereth!*

The Psalmist David made reference to the Lord first as the One "who forgiveth all thine iniquities," then as the One "who healeth all thy diseases" (Ps. 103:3).

Isaiah said of Jesus:

> But he was wounded **for our transgressions,** he was bruised **for our iniquities,** the chastisement of our peace was upon him; and with his stripes we are healed.
>
> Isaiah 53:5

If you don't know Jesus as the One who has washed your sins away and made you a new creature, then come to know Him today. (2 Cor. 5:17.) Right now!

> ...*if thou shalt confess with thy mouth the Lord Jesus, and shalt believe in thine heart that God hath raised him from the dead, thou shalt be saved.*
>
> Romans 10:9

Pray this prayer: *Jesus, I ask You into my heart as Lord and Savior of my life. Thank You for forgiving me of all my sins. I'm a new creature in You on the authority of Your Word. You're faithful to do what You said You would do if I would come to You and ask. Thank You, Jesus!*

Now that you're a child of God, if you need healing, you can come to the Father in Jesus' name and claim your healing. *You* can live and not die! *You* can talk to mountains. *You* can live a completely victorious life in Christ Jesus!

Prayer of Salvation

God loves you—no matter who you are, no matter what your past. God loves you so much that He gave His one and only begotten Son for you. The Bible tells us that "...whoever believes in him shall not perish but have eternal life" (John 3:16 NIV). Jesus laid down His life and rose again so that we could spend eternity with Him in heaven and experience His absolute best on earth. If you would like to receive Jesus into your life, say the following prayer out loud and mean it from your heart.

Heavenly Father, I come to You admitting that I am a sinner. Right now, I choose to turn away from sin, and I ask You to cleanse me of all unrighteousness. I believe that Your Son, Jesus, died on the cross to take away my sins. I also believe that He rose again from the dead so that I might be forgiven of my sins and made righteous through faith in Him. I call upon the name of Jesus Christ to be the Savior and Lord of my life. Jesus, I choose to follow You and ask that You fill me with the power of the Holy Spirit. I declare that right now I am a child of God. I am free from sin and full of the righteousness of God. I am saved in Jesus' name. Amen.

If you prayed this prayer to receive Jesus Christ as your Savior for the first time, please contact us on the Web at **www.harrisonhouse.com** to receive a free book.

Or you may write to us at
Harrison House
P.O. Box 35035
Tulsa, Oklahoma 74153

About the Author

Norvel Hayes shares God's Word boldly and simply with an enthusiasm that captures the heart of the hearer. He has learned through personal experience that God's Word can be effective in every area of life, and that it will work for anyone who will believe it and apply it.

Norvel owns several businesses which function successfully despite the fact that he spends over half his time away from the office, ministering the Gospel throughout the country. His obedience to God and his willingness to share his faith have taken him to a variety of places. He ministers in churches, seminars, conventions, colleges, prisons — anywhere the Spirit of God leads.

For a complete list of tapes and
books by Norvel Hayes, write:

Norvel Hayes
P O. Box 1379
Cleveland, TN 37311

Other Books by Norvel Hayes

Worship

The Blessing of Obedience

Confession Brings Possession

How To Get Your Prayers Answered

Let Not Your Heart Be Troubled

Misguided Faith

The Number One Way To Fight the Devil

What To Do for Healing

Why You Should Speak in Tongues

Additional copies of this book
are available from your local bookstore.

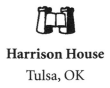

Harrison House
Tulsa, OK

www.harrisonhouse.com

Fast. Easy. Convenient!

- ◆ New Book Information
- ◆ Look Inside the Book
- ◆ Press Releases
- ◆ Bestsellers

- ◆ Free E-News
- ◆ Author Biographies
- ◆ Upcoming Books
- ◆ Share Your Testimony

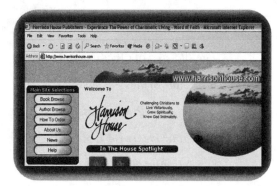

For the latest in book news and author information, please visit us on the Web at www.harrisonhouse.com. Get up-to-date pictures and details on all our powerful and life-changing products. Sign up for our e-mail newsletter, *Friends of the House,* and receive free monthly information on our authors and products including testimonials, author announcements, and more!

Harrison House—
Books That Bring Hope, Books That Bring Change

The Harrison House Vision

Proclaiming the truth and the power
Of the Gospel of Jesus Christ
With excellence;

Challenging Christians to
Live victoriously,
Grow spiritually,
Know God intimately.